PEDIATRIC EMERGENT/ URGENT AND AMBULATORY CARE

THE POCKET NP

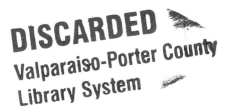

Sheila Sanning Shea, MSN, RN, ANP, is an emergency nurse practitioner (ENP) with over 40 years of clinical experience. She works in the Department of Emergency Medicine at St. Mary Medical Center, Long Beach, California. Ms. Shea established an emergency clinical fellowship for nurse practitioners and physician assistants that includes both didactic and clinical experiences. Ms. Shea is widely published and is an author and reviewer for the *Advanced Emergency Nursing Journal,* and was a contributing author to the *Emergency Nurses Core Curriculum* and *Certified Emergency Nurse Review.* Ms. Shea has taught NPs locally and nationally on a variety of emergent and urgent care topics.

Karen Sue Hoyt, PhD, RN, FNP-BC, ENP-C, FAEN, FAANP, FAAN, is an emergency nurse practitioner (ENP) and a professor and director of the NP/ENP programs at the Hahn School of Nursing and Health Science at the University of San Diego. Dr. Hoyt has several peer-reviewed books and publications on clinical practice, research, and management/leadership topics. In 2006, she established the first *Advanced Emergency Nursing Journal.* She conceptualized and has implemented a 2-day course for training ENPs and a train-the-trainer course for NP faculty. She has taught minor procedures workshops for NPs/PAs across the country. As a consultant and educator, she has also written ENP continuing education programs. Dr. Hoyt spearheaded *The Delphi Study on Competencies for NPs in Emergency Care* and serves as an item writer for the American Academy of Nurse Practitioners Certification Board. She is the former Chair of the NP Validation Committee for the American Academy of Emergency Nurse Practitioners.

Kathleen Sanders Jordan, DNP, RN, FNP-C, ENP-C, SANE-P, FAEN, FAANP, is currently a clinical associate professor in the Graduate School of Nursing at the University of North Carolina, Charlotte, North Carolina, teaching in the family nurse practitioner program and also in the DNP program. She is also employed as an emergency nurse practitioner with Mid-Atlantic Emergency Medical Associates in Charlotte and is the Advanced Practice Provider Fellowship Director. Dr. Jordan has been an advanced practice nurse in emergency care for over 35 years and is an examiner for the North Carolina Child Medical Evaluation Program. She is also a column editor for the *Advanced Emergency Nursing Journal.* She has published numerous articles and book chapters, has served as the lead editor for the *Core Curriculum for Emergency Nursing* for the Emergency Nurses Association, and currently serves as an item writer for the American Academy of Nurse Practitioners Certification Board.

PEDIATRIC EMERGENT/ URGENT AND AMBULATORY CARE

THE POCKET NP

SECOND EDITION

Sheila Sanning Shea, MSN, RN, ANP
Karen Sue Hoyt, PhD, RN, FNP-BC, ENP-C, FAEN,
    FAANP, FAAN
Kathleen Sanders Jordan, DNP, RN, FNP-C, ENP-C,
    SANE-P, FAEN, FAANP

SPRINGER PUBLISHING COMPANY

Springer Publishing Company, LLC
11 West 42nd Street, New York, NY 10036
www.springerpub.com
connect.springerpub.com/

Acquisitions Editor: Elizabeth Nieginski
Compositor: diacriTech

ISBN: 978-0-8261-5176-6
ebook ISBN: 978-0-8261-5177-3
DOI: 10.1891/9780826151773

20 21 22 23 / 5 4 3 2

The author and the publisher of this Work have made every effort to use sources believed to be reliable to provide information that is accurate and compatible with the standards generally accepted at the time of publication. Because medical science is continually advancing, our knowledge base continues to expand. Therefore, as new information becomes available, changes in procedures become necessary. We recommend that the reader always consult current research and specific institutional policies before performing any clinical procedure or delivering any medication. The author and publisher shall not be liable for any special, consequential, or exemplary damages resulting, in whole or in part, from the readers' use of, or reliance on, the information contained in this book. The publisher has no responsibility for the persistence or accuracy of URLs for external or third-party Internet websites referred to in this publication and does not guarantee that any content on such websites is, or will remain, accurate or appropriate.

Library of Congress Cataloging-in-Publication Data
Library of Congress Control Number: 2020902201

Sheila Sanning Shea: https://orcid.org/0000-0001-9163-7653
Karen Sue Hoyt: https://orcid.org/0000-0003-4810-2308
Kathleen Sanders Jordan: https://orcid.org/0000-0001-6011-5799

Publisher's Note: New and used products purchased from third-party sellers are not guaranteed for quality, authenticity, or access to any included digital components.

Printed in the United States of America.

CONTENTS

PREFACE

Pediatric Emergent/Urgent and Ambulatory Care: The Pocket NP is the result of three decades of our experiences as emergency nurse practitioners (ENPs). We often found our pockets filled with scribbled notes that included tidbits of things "not to miss," important "tips to remember," and essential information to include in the history and physical documentation. Although we had many excellent medical reference textbooks, we identified the need for a quick reference guide that had an easy-to-use framework for the most commonly encountered problems seen in the emergency, medical screening, fast-track, and/or primary care settings.

The guide focuses on the care of the pediatric patient and is arranged in a logical head-to-toe format that includes the history and physical examination, as well as essential medical decision-making considerations. Templates for "Dictation/Documentation" are provided to assist the clinician with the development of a concise and logical patient record. Also included are frequently used illustrations for anatomical reference.

HOW TO USE THIS GUIDE

Use appropriate sections of the "Pediatric Medical" or "Pediatric Trauma" template defaults to document basic normal findings. Delete any portion of the template that was not examined or is not pertinent to a specific patient. Mix and match portions of various templates to meet your needs and the components of the physical exam.

Fine-tune your assessment skills using the specific dictation/documentation templates for focused patient problems such as "knee pain."

Demonstrate your critical thinking skills by expanding and polishing your "Medical Decision-Making."

"Dictation/Documentation Guidelines" are designed as an outline to ensure that all critical elements of the patient record are addressed.

This guide is just that—a guide. It is intended as a quick reference tool only and it is not meant to be a complete review or definitive guide to clinical practice and patient management. The management options are based on current evidence for best practices. However, emergency medicine is an ever-changing specialty and the user of this guide is encouraged to consult other sources to confirm all medication indications, contraindications, side effects, and dosing prior to administration. The authors and the publisher specifically disclaim any liability for errors or omissions found here within, or for any misuse or treatment errors.

Sheila Sanning Shea
Karen Sue Hoyt

ABBREVIATIONS*

AB	Abortion
ABC	Airway breathing circulation
Abd	Abdomen/abdominal
ABG	Arterial blood gas
ABO	Blood type groups
Abx	Antibiotics
A-C	Acromioclavicular
ACL	Anterior cruciate ligament
ACS	Acute chest syndrome
ADL	Activities of daily living
AFib	Atrial fibrillation
AGE	Acute gastroenteritis
ALOC	Altered level of consciousness
ALTE	Apparent life-threatening event
AMS	Altered mental status
ANUG	Acute necrotizing ulcerative colitis
A&O	Alert and oriented
AOE	Acute otitis externa
AOM	Acute otitis media
A/P	Anterior/posterior
APAP	acetyl-para-aminophenol
APD	Afferent pupillary defect
APGAR	Appearance, pulse, grimace, activity, respirations
Appy	Appendicitis
ASA	Acetylsalicylic acid/aspirin
Assoc	Associated
AT	Atraumatic
ATFL	Anterior talofibular ligament
AVM	Arteriovenous malformation
AVN	Avascular necrosis
B-hCG	Beta human chorionic gonadotropin
BID	Twice a day
BM	Bowel movement
BMI	Body mass index
BMP	Basic metabolic panel
BO	Bowel obstruction
B/P	Blood pressure
BPD	Bronchopulmonary dysplasia
BPV	Benign positional vertigo
BS	Bowel sounds
BSA	Bowel sounds active
BUN	Blood urea nitrogen
CA	Cancer
CAP	Community acquired pneumonia
CBC	Complete blood count
CC	Chief complaint
CF	Cystic fibrosis
CFL	Calcaneofibular ligament
CHD	Congenital heart disease
Chem	Chemistries
CHF	Congestive heart failure
CKD	Chronic kidney disease
CMS	Circulation/motor/sensation
CMT	Cervical motion tenderness
CMV	Cytomegalovirus
CN	Cranial nerves (I–XII)
C/O	Complains of
CP	Chest pain
CPT	Current procedural terminology
CPK-MB	Creatine phosphokinase-MB
CRF	Chronic renal failure
CRL	Crown rump length
CRP	C-reactive protein
C&S	Culture and sensitivity
CSF	Cerebrospinal fluid
CT	Computerized tomography
CTA	Clear to auscultation
CVA	Cerebral vascular accident
CVA/CVAT	Costovertebral angle/costovertebral angle tenderness
CVD	Cardiovascular disease
Cx	Culture
CXR	Chest x-ray
D&C	Dilation and curettage
D/C	Diarrhea/constipation
DDD	Degenerative disc disease
DDx	Differential diagnoses
DHE	Dihydroergotamine
DI	Diabetes insipidus
DIC	Disseminated intravascular coagulopathy
DIP	Distal interphalangeal
DJD	Degenerative joint disease
DKA	Diabetic ketoacidosis
DM	Diabetes mellitus
DPT	Diphtheria pertussis tetanus
DS	Double strength
DSD	Dry sterile dressing
DTRs	Deep tendon reflexes
DVT	Deep vein thrombosis
Dxs	Diagnoses
EDC	Estimated date of confinement
EGD	Esophagogastroduodenoscopy
EH	Epidural hematoma
EKG	Electrocardiogram
E/M	Evaluation and management

*The abbreviations used in this book may not be accepted medical abbreviations.

EMLA	Lidocaine and prilocaine cream	HHS	Hyperosmolar hyperglycemic state
ENT	Ear, nose, and throat	HIV	Human immunodeficiency virus
EOM/EOMI	Extra ocular movements/extra ocular movements intact	HM	Hand motion
ESR	Erythrocyte sedimentation rate	HOB	Head of bed
		H&P	History and physical
ETOH	Ethanol (alcohol)	HPF	High powered field
Exac	Exacerbation	HPI	History of present illness
Extrems	Extremities	hr	Hour
FABER	Flexion, abduction, external rotation	HSM	Hepatosplenomegaly
		HSP	Henoch–Schonlein purpura
FAST	Focused assessment of sonography in trauma	HSV	Herpes simplex virus
		HTN	Hypertension
FB	Foreign body	HX	History
FBS	Fasting blood sugar	HZV	Herpes zoster virus
F/C	Fever/chills	IBD/IBS	Inflammatory bowel disease/ irritable bowel syndrome
FDP	Flexor digitorum profundus		
FDS	Flexor digitorum superficialis	ICH	Intracranial hemorrhage
		I&D	Incision and drainage
FH	Family history	IM	Intramuscular
FHCS	Fitz-Hugh–Curtis syndrome	Inj	Injury
FHM	Fetal heart motion/movement	Inpt	Inpatient
FI	Fecal incontinence	IO	Inferior oblique
FOOSH	Fall on outstretched hand	IO	Intraosseous
FROM	Full range of motion	IOP	Intraocular pressure
FSBS/FSBG	Finger stick blood sugar/ glucose	IR	Inferior rectus
		ITP	Idiopathic thrombocytopenic purpura
FTC	Full to confrontation		
F/U	Follow-up	IUP	Intrauterine pregnancy
FX	Fracture	IV	Intravenous
G	Gravida	IVDA	Intravenous drug abuse
GB	Gallbladder	IVF	In vitro fertilization
GC	Gonococcal/gonorrhea	IVIG	Intravenous immunoglobulin
GCS	Glasgow Coma Scale	JIA	Juvenile idiopathic arthritis
GERD	Gastroesophageal reflux disease	JLT	Joint like tenderness
		JVD	Jugular venous distention
GI	Gastrointestinal	K+	Potassium
GSW	Gunshot wound	KUB	Kidneys, ureters, bladder
Gtts	Drops	L	Left
GU	Genitourinary	l	Liter
GYN	Gynecologic	LCL	Lateral collateral ligament
HA	Headache	LDH	Lactate dehydrogenase
HbS	Hemoglobin S	LFT	Liver function tests
HCG	Human chorionic gonadotropin	LLQ	Left lower quadrant
		LMWH	Low molecular weight heparin
HEADSS	Home, education/ employment, activities, drugs, sexuality, suicide/depression	LNMP	Last normal menstrual period
		LOC	Loss of consciousness
		LP	Lumbar puncture
HEENT	Head/eyes/ears/nose/throat	LR	Lateral rectus
Heme	Hematologic	LSD	Lysergic acid diethylamide
Hep	Hepatitis	LSpine	Lumbosacral spine
HgbA1c	Hemoglobin A1c/ glycohemoglobin (for DM)	LUQ	Left upper quadrant
		LVF	Left ventricular failure

MAOIs	Monoamine oxidase inhibitors
MC	Metacarpal
MCL	Medial collateral ligament
MDM	Medical decision-making
Meds	Medications
MMM	Mucous membranes moist
MMR	Measles mumps rubella
MOI	Mechanism of injury
MR	Medial rectus
MRI	Magnetic resonance imaging
MRN	Medical record number
MRSA	Methicillin-resistant *Staphylococcus aureus*
MSK	Musculoskeletal
MTBI	Mild traumatic brain injury
MTPJ	Metatarsal phalangeal joint
MVC	Motor vehicle crash
NAAT	Nucleic acid amplification testing
NAD	No acute distress
NEXUS	National emergency x-radiology utilization study
NLP	No light perception
NPO	Nothing by mouth
NS	Normal saline
NSAIDs	Nonsteroidal anti-inflammatory drugs
NT	Nontender
N/V	Nausea/vomiting
N/V/D	Nausea/vomiting/diarrhea
NWB	Nonweight bearing
O₂Sat	Oxygen saturation/pulse oximetry
OB	Occult blood
OD	Overdose
OLDCART	Onset, location, duration, characteristics, aggravating factors, relieving factors, treatment
OME	Otitis media with effusion
Onc	Oncology
O&P	Ova and parasites
ORIF	Open reduction internal fixation
ORS	Oral rehydration solution
OTC	Over-the-counter
Outpts	Outpatients
P	Para
Palp	Palpate/palpitations
PCL	Posterior cruciate ligament
PCN	Penicillin
PCP	Phencyclidine
PCR	Polymerase chain reaction

PE	Pulmonary edema
PEx	Physical exam
Ped	Pediatric
PGE1	Prostaglandin E1
PERRLA	Pupils equal and round, reactive to light and accommodation
PID	Pelvic inflammatory disease
PIP	Proximal interphalangeal
PMD	Primary medical doctor
PMH	Past medical history
PNA	Pneumonia
PND	Paroxysmal nocturnal dyspnea
PO	Per os (by mouth)
POC	Products of conception
POF	Position of function
PPI	Proton pump inhibitor
PR	Per rectum
PRBCs	Packed red blood cells
PRN	As needed
prob	Problem
PSH	Past surgical history
Pt/Pts	Patient/Patients
PT	Point tenderness
PTFL	Posterior talofibular ligament
PUD	Peptic ulcer disease
PVK	Penicillin V potassium
PWD	Pink/warm/dry
QID	Four times per day
R	Right
RA	Rheumatoid arthritis
RBC	Red blood cell
Rh	Rhesus factor
RICE	Rest/ice/compression/elevation
RLQ	Right lower quadrant
RMSF	Rocky mountain spotted fever
R/O	Rule/out
ROM	Range of motion
ROS	Review of systems
RPR	Rapid plasma reagin
RRR	Regular rate and rhythm
RSV	Respiratory syncytial virus
RUQ	Right upper quadrant
SaO₂	Oxygen saturation (pulse oximetry)
SAB	Spontaneous abortion
SAH	Subarachnoid hemorrhage
SANE	Sexual assault response nurse
SBI	Serious bacterial infection
SBO	Small bowel obstruction
SCD	Sickle cell disease

SCFE	Slipped capital femoral epiphysis	tDAP	Tetanus diphtheria acellular pertussis
SCIWORA	Spinal cord injury without radiologic abnormality	TEN	Toxic epidermal necrolysis
SCM	Sternocleidomastoid	TENS	Transcutaneous electrical nerve stimulation
SH	Social history	TFL	Talofibular ligament
SH	Subdural hematoma	TID	Three times per day
SH	Surgical history	TM	Tympanic membrane
SI	Sciatic	TMJ	Temporomandibular joint
SIADH	Syndrome of inappropriate antidiuretic hormone	TMP/SMX	Trimethoprim (TMP) sulfamethoxazole (SMX)
SJS	Stevens–Johnson syndrome	TOA	Tubo-ovarian abscess
sle	Slit lamp exam	TPN	Total parenteral nutrition
SLE	Systemic lupus erythematosus	T&S	Type and screen
SLR	Straight leg raise	TSH	Thyroid stimulating hormone
SLUDGE	Salivation, lacrimation, diaphoresis/diarrhea, gastrointestinal cramping pain, emesis	TSS	Toxic shock syndrome
		TTP	Tender to palpation
		TV	Tidal volume
		UA	Urinalysis
SMR	Sexual maturity rating (Tanner staging)	UCG	Urine chorionic gonadotropin (Pregnancy test)
SNT	Soft, nontender	UCx	Urine culture
SO	Superior oblique	UI	Urinary incontinence
SOB	Shortness of breath	Ultz	Ultrasound
SR	Superior rectus	UOP	Urine output
SSS	Scalded skin syndrome	URI	Upper respiratory infection
SSSS	Staphylococcus	UTI	Urinary tract infection
STEMI	ST elevation myocardial infarction	Utox	Urine toxicology
		V/A	Visual/acuity
STI	Sexually transmitted infection	V/D	Vomiting/diarrhea
STS	Soft tissue swelling	VBG	Venous blood gas
SubQ	Subcutaneous	V/F	Visual fields
SXS	Symptoms	VP	Ventriculoperitoneal
TAB	Therapeutic abortion	VS	Vital signs
TAD	Thoracic aortic dissection	VSS	Vital signs stable
TB	Tuberculosis	WBC	White blood count
TBI	Traumatic brain injury	WDWN	Well-developed, well-nourished
TBSA	Total body surface area	WNL	Within normal limits
T&C	Type and crossmatch	WOB	Work of breathing
TCA	Tricyclic antidepressants	X-ray	Radiographic

DICTATION/DOCUMENTATION GUIDELINES

HPI

Based on chief complaint, OLD CART:

- O—Onset
- L—Location
- D—Duration
- C—Characteristics
- A—Aggravating factors
- R—Relieving factors
- T—Treatment

PAST MEDICAL HISTORY

Infants: perinatal and neonatal history: term birth, birth weight, vaginal versus cesarean, complications during pregnancy, labor, and/or delivery, APGAR, perinatal exposure of infections, feeding patterns, mother's strep B status treated (important for neonatal sepsis), mother immunized in third trimester for pertussis?

PREVIOUS ILLNESSES, HOSPITALIZATIONS, AND SURGERIES
ALLERGIES/IMMUNIZATIONS
FAMILY/SOCIAL HISTORY (INCLUDE DEVELOPMENTAL MILESTONES)
REVIEW OF SYSTEMS
PHYSICAL EXAMINATION

VITAL SIGNS

Note vital signs and interpret as normal or abnormal for age (include blood pressure [BP] for >3 years old). Note weight in kg and body mass index (BMI)

GENERAL

Patient (pt) is well developed, well nourished, and in no acute distress (NAD). Patient is awake, alert, and interactive, with behavior appropriate for age. Dressed appropriately and well kempt

SKIN

Intact, pink, warm, dry. Good turgor without tenting. No rash, ecchymosis, or edema

HEENT

- **Head:** normocephalic, atraumatic. Anterior fontanel soft and flat
- **Eyes:** sclera clear and moist and conjunctiva pink. No discharge. PERRLA (pupils equal and round, reactive to light and accommodation). EOMI (extra ocular movements/ extra ocular movements intact) without strabismus. Gross visual acuity intact. Fundi unable to visualize, positive red reflex bilaterally
- **Ears:** pinna is normal shape and contour. Clear external auditory canals. Tympanic membrane pearly gray with good cone of light, no erythema or suppuration. No pre- or postauricular adenopathy. No gross hearing deficit
- **Nose:** pink, moist mucosa with good air movement. No rhinorrhea or nasal flaring. Septum midline
- **Mouth:** moist mucous membranes. Good dentition without caries or gingival hypertrophy
- **Throat:** posterior pharynx pink and moist without erythema, exudate, or ulceration. Uvula midline. Normal movement of soft palate

(cont.)

DICTATION/DOCUMENTATION GUIDELINES (cont.)

NECK
Supple with normal range of motion (ROM). No edema or tracheal deviation. No lymphadenopathy, goiter, or masses

CHEST
Sexual maturity rating. Chest moves symmetrically without increased work of breathing, retractions, or use of accessory muscles. Lungs CTA (clear to auscultation) with no stridor, crackles, wheezes, or rhonchi

HEART
No heaves. RRR (regular rate and rhythm). Positive S1, S2, negative S3, S4, without murmurs, rubs, or gallops. Distal pulses symmetric. Capillary refill <2 seconds

ABDOMEN
Not distended. Bowel sounds present. Soft, nontender, no palpable masses. No hepato-splenomegaly or CVAT (costovertebral angle/costovertebral angle tenderness)

BACK
FROM, nontender, no lordosis or kyphosis

GU (GENITOURINARY)
Sexual maturity rating. Female: external genitalia, vulva, hymen shape, no vaginal discharge. Male: circumcised, testes descended bilaterally, cremasteric reflex present bilaterally

EXTREMITIES
Symmetric without deformity, warm. No clubbing, cyanosis, or edema. Negative Barlow and Ortolani signs

NEURO
Mental status: affect. LOC (loss of consciousness), speech. Motor: normal gait, muscle strength, and tone for developmental level. CN II-XII intact, DTRs (deep tendon reflexes) 2+/2+ bilaterally. No meningeal signs

MEDICAL TEMPLATE

GENERAL

The pt is a well-developed, well-nourished child who is awake and active. Interacts appropriately with surroundings and examiner, in no acute distress

VITAL SIGNS

Note VS and interpret as normal or abnormal, SaO_2 interpretation, weight in kg

SKIN

Pink, warm, and dry. Normal texture and turgor without rash or cyanosis

HEENT

- **Head:** normocephalic without evidence of trauma. Fontanel normal (if still open)
- **Eyes:** moist and bright. Sclera and conjunctivae normal. Pupils are equal, round, and reactive to light. Extraocular movements intact. No nystagmus or diplopia noted
- **Ears:** canals patent. Tympanic membranes clear. No pre- or postauricular lymphadenopathy
- **Nose:** patent without rhinorrhea or nasal flaring
- **Mouth/Throat:** mucous membranes moist. Posterior pharynx clear without lesions, erythema, or exudates

NECK

Full ROM. Supple without meningismus or lymphadenopathy

CHEST

No retractions noted; no grunting or stridor. Good tidal volume. Lungs clear to auscultation; no wheezes, rales, or rhonchi. SaO_2 ___%, which is within normal limits (if 95% or >)

HEART

Tones normal. RRR. No murmurs, rubs, or gallops are heard

ABDOMEN

Soft, nondistended. Bowel sounds are active. No apparent tenderness. No masses or organomegaly palpated

BACK

Without spinal or CVA tenderness

GU

Normal external genitalia without rash. No hernia noted

EXTREMITIES

Full ROM. Good strength bilaterally. Neurovascular intact. No cyanosis or edema

NEURO

Alert, active, and developmentally normal for age. GCS 15 4/6/5. Muscle tone good and equal, bilaterally. No focal neurological findings noted

TRAUMA TEMPLATE

GENERAL
The pt is well developed. Awake, alert, and conversant in no apparent distress

VITAL SIGNS
Note VS and interpret as normal or abnormal, pulse ox interpretation, weight in kg

SKIN
Warm and dry, intact

HEENT
- **Head:** normocephalic atraumatic without palpable deformities
- **Eyes:** pupils equal, round, and reactive to light. Extraocular movements intact. No periorbital ecchymosis or step-off
- **Ears:** canals patent. Tympanic membranes are clear. No Battle's sign. No hemotympanum
- **Nose/Face:** atraumatic. There is no septal hematoma. Facial bones are nontender to palpation and stable with attempts at manipulation
- **Mouth/Throat:** no intraoral trauma. Teeth and mandible are intact

NECK
No midline point tenderness, step-off, or deformity to firm palpation of posterior cervical spine. Trachea midline. Carotids equal (2+/2+). No masses. No JVD. Full ROM of the neck without limitation or pain

CHEST
No surface trauma. Nontender without crepitus or deformity. No palpable subcutaneous air. Lungs have good tidal volume with normal breath sounds bilaterally

HEART
Regular rate and rhythm. Tones are normal and clear

ABDOMEN
No abrasions, ecchymosis, or surface trauma. Bowel sounds are active. No distention. Nontender to palpation; no guarding, rebound, or rigidity. No masses

BACK
No contusions, ecchymosis, or abrasions are noted. Nontender without step-off or deformity to firm midline palpation. No CVAT or flank ecchymosis

GU
Normal external genitalia with no blood at the meatus. No scrotal swelling or tenderness

PELVIS
Nontender to palpation and stable to compression. Femoral pulses strong and equal (2+/2+)

RECTAL
Normal tone. No rectal wall tenderness or mass. Stool is brown and heme negative

EXTREMITIES
No surface trauma. Full ROM without limitation or pain. Good strength in all extremities. Sensation to light touch intact. All peripheral pulses are intact and equal

NEURO
A&O × 3, GCS 15 4/6/5, CN II–XII intact. Motor and sensory exam nonfocal. Reflexes are symmetric.

REVIEW OF SYSTEMS

Usually abbreviated for infants and younger children. If pertinent to the chief complaint include: prenatal and birth history, developmental history, social history of family, environmental risks, and immunization history

GENERAL
Birth weight, weight changes, appetite change, fever, chills, changes in behavior or activity level

DERM
Rashes, itching, exposure to rashes, adenopathy, lumps, bruising and bleeding, pigmentation changes

NEURO
Change in mental status, behavior changes, dizziness, HA, seizures, weakness, ataxia, concentration, syncope, breath holding spells, history of head trauma

HEENT
Unusual head shape, concussions, visual problems, eye redness/drainage, ear infections, ear drainage, hearing, sore throats, nasal congestion, allergies, epistaxis, snoring, sore throats, difficulty swallowing or drooling, caries, last dental exam

CV
Murmurs, exercise tolerance, cyanosis, chest pain, palpitations

RESP
Wheezing, cough, dyspnea, pneumonia, bronchiolitis

GI
Appetite, feeding pattern, stool color and character, diarrhea, constipation, vomiting, abd pain, jaundice, colic

GU
Patterns, independent, dysuria, frequency, urgency, hematuria, polyuria, enuresis, vaginal discharge, penile discharge, testicular pain/swelling

PUBERTAL
Secondary sexual characteristics, menarche, LNMP (last normal menstrual period), pregnancies, sexual activity

MUSCULOSKELETAL
Limp, gait change, pain or swelling, injuries

ENDOCRINE
Polyuria, polydipsia, hair or skin changes, parental concern regarding rate of growth, age of puberty

PSYCH
Depression, self-mutilation, anxiety, anger, aggression, suicidal/homicidal ideation

ALLERGIES/IMMUNIZATION
Urticarial, rhinitis, asthma, eczema, drug reactions, immunization status

BILLING CONSIDERATIONS

Level 1	Level 2–3	Level 4 or 5
Problem Focused	Expanded Problem Focused	Detailed or Comprehensive
Chief complaint	Chief complaint	Chief complaint
HPI: Focused 1–3 elements	HPI: 1–3 elements	HPI: >4 elements or status of three or more chronic or inactive conditions
PMH: None required	PMH	PMH
FH/SH: None required	FH/SH: None required, include if pertinent	FH/SH: Detailed
ROS: None required	ROS: 1 element	ROS: 2–10 elements
Exam: Focused exam of one body area or organ system	Exam: Focused exam of one body area or organ system plus related organ system or symptom	Exam: Detailed and comprehensive
MDM: Minimal number of diagnostic or treatment options Minimal or no data reviewed Minimal risk complications, morbidity, or mortality	MDM: Limited number of diagnostic or treatment options Limited or no data reviewed Limited risk complications, morbidity, or mortality (Difference in level 2 or 3 depends on complexity of decision-making such as consideration of differential diagnoses.)	MDM: Highly complex and detailed

Current Procedural Terminology (CPT) and Evaluation and Management (E/M) codes are for nongovernmental payers and are the insurance industry standard. Levels of care range from 1 to 5; in order to score a chart for billing, a certain level of care and varying numbers of organ systems must be reviewed. Claims submitted to Medicaid and/or Medicare for services provided for pediatric pts must adhere to the Centers for Medicare B & Medicaid Services Documentation Guidelines for Evaluation and Management Services.

NEONATAL JAUNDICE

HX

- Yellowish face, sclera, trunk
- Breast or bottle-fed; adequacy of nursing or taking a bottle
- Weak suck, latching problems, milk output, breast engorgement, duration of nursing
- High-pitched cry, lethargy, change in muscle tone, seizure
- Pre- and postnatal history
    - Adjusted or corrected age if preterm <38 weeks
- Urine and stool output, loss of stool color
- Birthweight, current wt, >10% wt loss is concerning in newborn
- Delivery HX: delayed cord clamping, birth trauma with bruising and/or FXs
- Maternal OB HX: maternal illness, illicit drug use
- SXS/signs: hypothyroidism, metabolic disease (e.g., galactosemia), recent TPN
- FH: sibling with HX jaundice, blood group incompatibility, hemolysis, phototherapy, or exchange transfusion
- Gilbert syndrome anemia, splenectomy, bile stones in family members or known heredity for hemolytic disorders, liver disease
- Blood type, DM, ethnicity

PE

- **General:** WDWN infant, awake, and active. Interacts appropriately with surroundings and examiner, in no acute distress. No drowsiness or lethargy
- **VS and SaO$_2$**
- **Skin:** jaundice of forehead and face; emphasized by pressure, trunk, and/or extremities (jaundice moves from head to toe and corresponds to total bilirubin: face 5 mg/dL; 15 mg/dL mid-abd; jaundice resolves in opposite direction) or skin PWD; normal texture and turgor without rash, cyanosis, or petechiae
- **HEENT:**
    - **Head:** normocephalic without evidence of trauma. Fontanel normal.
    - **Eyes:** moist and bright. Sclera and conjunctivae normal or icteric. PERRL. EOMIs
    - **Ears:** canals patent. Tympanic membranes clear
    - **Nose:** patent without rhinorrhea or nasal flaring
    - **Mouth/Throat:** mucous membranes moist. Posterior pharynx clear without lesions, erythema, or exudates
- **Neck:** supple, no meningismus or lymphadenopathy
- **Chest:** no retractions noted; no grunting or stridor. Good tidal volume. Lungs CTA; no wheezes, crackles, or rhonchi. SaO$_2$ ___%, which is within normal limits
- **Heart:** RRR, no murmurs, rubs, or gallops
- **Abd:** soft, nondistended. No apparent tenderness. No masses or organomegaly palpated. BSA
- **Back:** without spinal or CVA tenderness
- **GU:** normal external genitalia without rash. No hernia noted
- **Extremities**: good muscle tone, moves all extremities, neurovascular intact
- **Neuro:** alert and developmentally normal for age. Muscle tone good and equal, bilaterally. No focal neurological findings noted

(cont.)

NEONATAL JAUNDICE (cont.)

MDM/DDx

Jaundice is the most common condition that requires medical management in neonates. Yellowish skin and sclera results from accumulation of unconjugated bilirubin. Normal or **physiologic jaundice** (unconjugated hyperbilirubinemia) is caused by the neonate's immature liver and inability to process bilirubin. Physiologic jaundice peaks at 3 to 5 days in bottle-fed infants and usually resolves spontaneously by 7 days. **Breast milk jaundice** can last up to 3 weeks. Bilirubin is neurotoxic and severe hyperbilirubinemia can cause brain damage **(kernicterus)** or even death. MDM is directed to prevention of neurotoxicity and identification of the pathologic causes of jaundice such as occult infection. Consider **galactosemia** or **congenital hypothyroidism** for severe or persistent jaundice >1 to 2 weeks. Hepatosplenomegaly, petechiae, and microcephaly may be associated with **hemolytic anemia, sepsis**, and **congenital infections** such as CMV. Other potential causes for jaundice include **cholestasis** (with use of TPN), **duodenal atresia, and neonatal hepatitis syndrome**

MANAGEMENT

LABS

- ▨ Well-appearing 2- to 3-day-old neonate with jaundice: total bilirubin level only
- ▨ Bilirubin fractions are not indicated: indirect = unconjugated; direct = conjugated
- ▨ Ill-appearing with jaundice on day 1 of life or neonate >3 days with jaundice
- ▨ CBC with differential, chemistry panel, total bilirubin, direct (Coombs) and indirect bilirubin, type and Rh (mother and child), serum albumin, reticulocyte count, LFTs, UA. Possible ABG/VBG, thyroid function tests

IMAGING

- ▨ Ultz liver and bile ducts: if cholestatic Dx suspected; radionuclide liver scan: if extrahepatic biliary atresia suspected

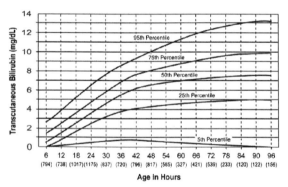

Nomogram showing smoothed curves for the 5th, 25th, 50th, 75th, and 95th percentiles for transcutaneous bilirubin (TcB) measurements among healthy newborns (gestational age ≥35 weeks)

Source: Reproduced with permission from Maisels, M. J., DeRidder, J. M., Kring, J. E. A., & Balasubramaniam, M. (2009). Routine transcutaneous bilirubin measurements combined with clinical risk factors improve the prediction of subsequent hyperbilirubinemia. *Journal of Perinatology, 29*(1), 612–617. Figure 1.

(cont.)

NEONATAL JAUNDICE (cont.)

OTHER PHOTOTHERAPY
- IVIG
- Exchange transfusion for severe cases to prevent neurotoxicity
- GI consult if hepatobiliary or bowel disease

DICTATION/DOCUMENTATION
- **General:** WDWN neonate who is awake and active. Interacts appropriately with surroundings and examiner, in no acute distress
- **VS and SaO$_2$:** note VS and interpret as normal or abnormal, SaO$_2$ interpretation, weight in kg
- **Skin:** jaundiced, or pink, warm, and dry. Normal texture and turgor without rash or cyanosis.
- **HEENT:**
  - **Head:** normocephalic without evidence of trauma. Fontanel normal.
  - **Eyes:** moist and bright. Sclera and conjunctivae normal. PERRLA. EOMIs
  - **Ears:** canals patent. Tympanic membranes clear. No pre- or postauricular lymphadenopathy
  - **Nose:** patent without rhinorrhea or nasal flaring
  - **Mouth/Throat:** mucous membranes moist. Posterior pharynx clear without lesions, erythema, or exudates
- **Neck:** full range of motion. Supple without meningismus or lymphadenopathy
- **Chest:** no retractions noted; no grunting or stridor. Good tidal volume. CTA; no wheezes, crackles, or rhonchi. SaO$_2$ ___%, which is within normal limits (if 95% or >)
- **Heart:** RRR, no murmurs, rubs, or gallops are heard
- **Abd:** soft, BSA, nondistended. No apparent tenderness. No masses or organomegaly palpated
- **Back:** without spinal or CVAT
- **GU:** normal external genitalia without rash. No hernia noted
- **Extremities:** FROM. Good strength bilaterally. Neurovascular intact. No cyanosis or edema
- **Neuro:** alert, active, and developmentally normal for age. GCS 15. Muscle tone good and equal, bilaterally. No focal neurological findings noted

○ TIPS
- Signs of neonatal jaundice
- Birth wt versus current wt, >10% wt loss is concerning in newborn delivery HX: delayed cord clamping, birth trauma with bruising and/or FXs, maternal illnesses, illicit drug use
- FH: Sibling with neonatal jaundice, blood group incompatibility, hemolysis, phototherapy, or exchange transfusion

DON'T MISS!
- Ill-appearing jaundiced infants should have immediate phototherapy while workup is initiated

SKIN RASHES/LESIONS

HX

- Appearance
- OLDCART: Onset, Location (distribution and progression), Duration, Characteristics (e.g., pruritic, burning), Aggravating or Relieving factors, and Treatments employed prior to arrival
- Mucous membrane involvement, palmer/sole involvement
- Quality: painful, paresthesias
- Associated symptoms: signs of systemic illness, fever, chills, headache, sore throat, myalgias, arthralgias, wheezing, edema, coryza
- Possible exposures (e.g., medication, personal care products, recreation, travel, food)
- Other contacts with similar symptoms
- Past medical history
- Allergies

PE

- **General:** awake, alert, age-appropriate behavior, well versus toxic appearing
- **VS and SaO$_2$:** note if febrile
- **Skin:**
    - **Primary lesion:** macule, papule, plaque, nodule, wheal, vesicle, pustule, bullae, cyst, or ulcer. **Secondary lesion:** excoriation, edema, scale, crust, fissure, erosion, indurated, fluctuant, atrophy, scar, hypopigmentation
    - **Location/Distribution:** generalized, localized, dermatomal, discrete, diffuse, confluent, grouped, annular, linear, discoid
    - Color/temperature: erythema, blanching, warm/hot
- **HEENT:**
    - **Head:** normocephalic, atraumatic, kerion, scaly patches, hair loss
    - **Eyes:** PERRLA, EOMI, sclera and conjunctiva clear, periorbital lesions, STS, or erythema
    - **Ears:** canals and TMs normal, pre- or postauricular lymphadenopathy
    - **Nose:** normal, rhinorrhea. Vesicle at tip of nose (Hutchinson sign) concern for ophthalmic HZV.
    - **Face:** symmetric, "slapped cheeks" lesions
    - **Mouth/Throat:** MMM; dry, cracked lips; posterior pharynx clear; mucosal lesions; strawberry tongue; palatine petechiae; vesicles; Koplik spots
- **Neck:** supple, FROM, lymphadenopathy, or meningismus
- **Chest:** CTA, heart sounds
- **Abd:** soft, NT, BSA, no HSM
- **Back:** spinal or CVAT
- **Extremities:** FROM with good strength

(cont.)

SKIN RASHES/LESIONS (cont.)

MDM/DDx

Life-threatening: primary goal is to identify and treat rashes that represent serious or life-threatening disease. Most acute, urgent rashes are *erythematous. Rashes associated with fever and hypotension* include TSS (staph variant), **RMSF, and meningococcal infections.** *Erythematous rash with signs of systemic illness:* **enterovirus** (maculopapular, vesicular, urticarial rash), **erythema infectiosum (fifth disease, slapped cheek syndrome),** roseola (faint, maculopapular rash 2–3 days after fever), scarlet fever (sandpaper, blanches). **Vesiculopustular rash:** *impetigo* (honey crusting), **SSS,** generalized erythema, Nikolsky's sign, **HSV** (grouped thick-walled vesicles and pustules), HSZ (grouped papules, vesicles, erosions), **erythema multiforme** (papules, wheals, target lesions), **TEN; SJS** is a milder form of TEN: generalized erythema, sloughing, Nikolsky's sign. *Petechiae/Purpuricvious rash:* **ITP, HSP** on lower extremities, **acute leukemia (generalized),** and DIC. *Papulosquamous/ Eczematous rash:* **atopic dermatitis, diaper dermatitis (consider candida), allergic dermatitis** (red papules or vesicles), edema; **eczema herpeticum,** herpes clusters at site of eczema; **pityriasis rosea** (papules, scales in a Christmas-tree pattern), **tinea** (scales, papules, pustules, vesicles), **seborrheic dermatitis, cutis marmorata, intertrigo, Type IV hypersensitivity reaction, syphilis, vasculitis.** *Others:* **scabies** (pruritic, excoriated papules, skin burrows, interdigital spaces), **Kawasaki disease** (fever; conjunctivitis; strawberry tongue; dry, cracked lips; erythema of palms and soles; polymorphous truncal rash; cervical adenopathy). *Neonatal rash:* **benign pustular dermatoses** (macules and papules evolve to pustules), **milia** (pearly, yellow papules on face), **candida, seborrheic dermatitis** (yellow scales on intertriginous areas and scalp). *Serious neonatal rashes* include **congenital syphilis** (maculopapular rash with systemic illness), **herpes simplex** (clustered papules and vesicles)

PRIMARY LESIONS

- **Macule:** less than 1 cm (over 1 cm is patch)
- **Papule:** solid raised lesion with distinct borders, <1 cm; may be domed, flat-topped, umbilicated
- **Nodule:** raised solid lesion more than 1 cm (mass >1 cm)
- **Plaque:** solid, raised, flat-topped (plateau) lesion >1 cm in diameter
- **Vesicle:** raised lesions <1 cm in diameter that are filled with clear fluid
- **Pustule:** circumscribed elevated pustular lesions commonly infected
- **Bullae:** circumscribed fluid-filled lesions that are >1 cm in diameter
- **Wheal:** area of edema in the upper epidermis
- **Burrow:** linear lesions produced by infestation of the skin and formation of tunnels

SECONDARY LESIONS

- **Excoriation:** abrasions that cause loss of epidermis, often linear
- **Crust:** dried exudate of serum, blood, or pus
- **Scale:** flaky white or skin-colored plates on the surface of the skin
- **Fissures:** linear cleavages on epidermis that can extend through the dermis, painful
- **Erosions/ulcers:** loss of all or part of epidermis/can extend through the dermis
- **Atrophy:** thinning or loss of epidermis and dermis, skin translucent, and depressed
- **Indurated:** hardened, loss of elasticity
- **Fluctuant:** moveable and compressible

(cont.)

SKIN RASHES/LESIONS (cont.)

MANAGEMENT

OTC topical ointments/creams can be used for minor skin infections (e.g., bacitracin, neosporin). Clarify all topical antifungals and oral antivirals. When early MRSA is suspected mupirocin (Bactroban 0.2%) applied BID to the affected area is recommended for 7 to 10 days. For more serious infections, oral, IM, IV abx will be used. Treatment with antibiotics will depend on the microorganism (e.g., antibacterials—clindamycin or Bactrim or Keflex for strep coverage). Refer to antibiogram/antibiotic policy at facility

DICTATION/DOCUMENTATION

- **General:** well appearing, nontoxic, age appropriate
- **VS and SaO$_2$:** afebrile
- **Skin:** color, temperature, moisture, texture, turgor. Note mucous membrane involvement, blisters, peeling, extensive erythema, presence or absence of purpura/petechiae, or secondary infection. Note whether palms and soles involved. Describe rash or lesions, including location, distribution, configuration

ALLERGIC REACTION/ANAPHYLAXIS MANAGEMENT

- Diphenhydramine 1 mg/kg not to exceed 50 mg/dose; PO for mild cases. Can also be given IM/IV
- Ranitidine 1 mg/kg (150 mg/dose PO for mild cases; not to exceed 50 mg/dose IV)
- Corticosteroids do not have an immediate effect on the SXS of anaphylaxis but may reduce/prevent a "late phase" reaction. Prednisone, prednisolone (PO) 1 to 2 mg/kg, or methylprednisolone (IV) admin is chosen based on the pt's clinical presentation. Dexamethasone 0.15 to 0.6 mg/kg IV can be given and dose repeated every 6 hours
- Epinephrine 1:1,000 IM in anterolateral thigh; may repeat every 5 to 15 minutes. SubQ administration no longer recommended. Because of the risk of potentially lethal dysrhythmias, IV/IO epinephrine (1:10,000) is reserved for the pt with uncompensated shock
- Nebulized albuterol (2.5–5 mg/dose) may be used for bronchospasm not responding to epinephrine
- Nebulized epinephrine has been used for stridor secondary to laryngeal edema
- IV with crystalloids or IO access when IV access cannot be quickly established in hemodynamically unstable pts
- Pts with hypotension unresponsive to modified Trendelenburg position and epinephrine should receive a 20 mL/kg rapid crystalloid fluid bolus (e.g., LR or NS)
- Repeat boluses up to 60 to 80 mL/kg may be necessary for correcting hypoperfusion secondary to vasodilatory shock

BURNS

HX

- MOI (maintain a high index of suspicion for nonaccidental trauma)
- Type of burn, length of exposure to the burn agent, falls, explosions, exposure to chemicals or electrical current
- Time of burn injury
- Possibility of inhalation injury (closed space exposure, carbon monoxide, cyanide)
- Concomitant trauma
- Past medical history
- Tetanus immunization status
- Allergies
- Risk for child maltreatment/interpersonal/family violence (see "Maltreatment")

PE

- **General:** level of pain and distress
- **VS and SaO$_2$**
- **Skin:** color, temperature, TBSA, circumferential burns (see "Tips"), depth of burn:
  - **Superficial (first degree):** epidermis only, red and painful, blanches with pressure
  - **Superficial partial thickness (second degree):** epidermis and superficial dermis, painful, red, weeping, blistered, blanches with pressure. May be a **deep partial thickness** (second degree) that is less painful, blisters, patchy red and white, wet to waxy dry, nonblanching
  - **Full thickness (third degree):** through epidermis and dermis, lack of sensation, waxy white to leathery gray to charred and black, dry and inelastic, nonblanching
- **HEENT:**
  - **Head:** atraumatic
  - **Eyes:** PERRLA, periorbital STS, erythema, singed lashes, scleral injection, corneal epithelial defect with fluorescein stain under Wood's lamp
  - **Ears:** TMs and canals normal, no STS or erythema
  - **Nose/Face:** singed nasal hairs, facial burns
  - **Mouth/Throat:** burned or swollen lips, drooling, stridor, dysphagia, odor of soot on breath, carbonaceous secretions, intraoral burns
- **Neck:** STS
- **Chest:** tachypnea, dyspnea, retractions, grunting, coughing, wheezing, rhonchi; surface burns
- **Heart:** RRR
- **Abd:** surface trauma, soft, BSA, nontender without guarding or rebound
- **Back:** no spinal or CVAT
- **Pelvis:** nontender to palpation; no erythema, STS, or burn of external genitalia
- **Extremities:** atraumatic, normal strength and tone, no STS, normal peripheral pulses in each limb
- **Neuro:** awake, alert, age-appropriate behavior

(cont.)

BURNS (cont.)

MDM/DDx

Inhalation and airway injuries are the most common cause of death in pediatric burn pts. Evidence of airway compromise and respiratory distress must be aggressively managed, often requiring early intubation. High-risk symptoms that may indicate the need for intubation include persistent cough, wheezing, or stridor; carbonaceous sputum or severe blistering in the oropharynx; severe facial burns; circumferential neck burns; altered mental status; respiratory distress; worsening hypoxia; or hypercapnia. Pediatric burn pts are at higher risk of developing dehydration and shock because of increased TBSA-to-volume ratio. Burns to critical areas, such as the face, hands, feet, genitalia, and across major joints, often require transfer to a burn center. **Consider the possibility of child maltreatment burns in all pediatric pts.** Index of suspicion should be high when there is an inconsistent history with the pattern of injury or the developmental level of the child, a delay in treatment of burns, discrete burn margins, lack of splash burns in scald injuries, unburned areas within the burned area (e.g., on buttocks), stocking-glove distribution, well-demarcated circular or point burns (e.g., cigarette), or concomitant bruising, FXs, or other trauma

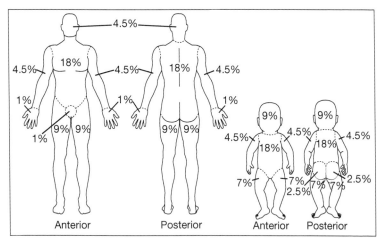

Rule of nines burn chart (adult and child)
Source: Reproduced from Veenema, T. G. (2019). *Disaster nursing and emergency preparedness: For chemical, biological, and radiological terrorism and other hazards* (4th ed.) New York, NY: Springer Publishing Company.

(cont.)

BURNS (cont.)

MANAGEMENT
Major Burns

- Immediate stabilization, ABCs, continuous pulse oximetry, O_2 administration, IV access
- **Fluid administration:** for burns that exceed 15% TBSA use the Parkland formula ($4 \times$ weight [kg] $\times$ % TBSA burn), administering lactated Ringer's solution (in children <20 kg D5LR should be used to support metabolic needs)
- Administer 50% fluid over the first 8 hours, and infuse the remaining fluid over the next 16 hours. Maintenance fluid must also be given concomitantly. Goal is to maintain urine output of 1 mL/kg per hour or more
- **Pain management:** Fentanyl (0.5–1.5 mcg/kg/dose IV or intranasal), morphine (0.1 mg/kg/dose IV or IM), toradol (0.5 mg/kg IV to a maximum of 15 mg)
- **Labs:** CBC with diff, chem panel, UA, urine myoglobin (suspected muscle injury), carboxyhemoglobin level (suspected inhalation injury), ABG
- **Burn care:** cover with a dry sterile dressing pending transfer to a burn center. Avoid wet dressings that exacerbate hypothermia
- **Imaging:** dictated by the presence of concomitant injury
- Monitor for rhabdomyolysis:
  - Myalgias
  - Generalized weakness
  - Darkened urine

Minor Burns

- **Pain management:** Tylenol with codeine (1 mg/kg/dose of codeine component), Lortab Elixir (0.1 mg/kg/dose of hydrocodone component), or acetaminophen alone (15 mg/kg/dose). Ibuprofen (10 mg/kg IV) is very effective in conjunction with opiates because of its anti-inflammatory effect
- **Burn care:** clean burns with mild soap and water; debride devitalized tissue; leave blisters intact; apply a simple antibiotic ointment (e.g., bacitracin, Silvadene), or apply a commercially prepared synthetic occlusive dressing; cover with nonadherent dressing and wrap with woven gauze bandage

CRITERIA FOR ADMISSION TO A BURN CENTER

- Partial thickness burns >20% TBSA at any age or >10% TBSA in those <10 years of age
- Full thickness burns > 5% TBSA
- Any significant burn to the face, hands, joints, genitalia, or perineum
- Inhalation, chemical, or electrical injury
- Significant associated injuries
- **Pts who do not meet these criteria should be admitted to an inpt pediatric unit if any of the following are present:**
  - Age <10 with 5%–10% TBSA affected
  - Age >10 with >10% TBSA affected
  - Inability to take PO fluids, full thickness burns
  - 2% TBSA; high voltage injuries, circumferential burns; suspected child maltreatment

(cont.)

BURNS (cont.)

DICTATION/DOCUMENTATION

- **General:** awake and alert, not toxic appearing
- **VS and SaO$_2$**
- **Skin:** estimated % TBSA of burn and method of calculation (e.g., Lund and Browder chart); depth and description of burns; presence of circumferential burns
- **HEENT:**
  - **Head:** atraumatic, nontender, fontanel flat
  - **Eyes:** sclera and conjunctiva clear, PERRLA, EOMI
  - **Ears:** TMs and canals clear
  - **Nose/Face:** no facial burn, nasal flare
  - **Mouth/Throat:** lips without burn or STS, no drooling, stridor, dysphagia, odor of soot on breath, carbonaceous secretions, intraoral burns MMM, posterior pharynx clear
- **Neck:** supple, FROM, no STS
- **Chest:** no surface burn, no retractions or accessory muscle use; CTA, no wheezing, rhonchi, crackles
- **Heart:** RRR, no murmurs, rubs, or gallops
- **Abd:** no surface burn, soft, BSA, NT
- **Extrems:** no surface burns, STS, FROM, good muscle strength and tone, pulses intact in all limbs

▶ TIP

- Palmar surface of the child's hand = ~1% of TBSA

DON'T MISS!

The characteristics of maltreatment:
- Location of the injury
- Pattern of the injury
- Consistency of the MOI and the presenting injury and developmental level of the child
- Degree or extent of the injury
- Delay in treatment of burns
- Discrete burn margins

- Lack of splash burns in scald injuries
- Nonburned areas within the burn region (e.g., on buttocks), stocking-glove distribution, well-demarcated circular or point burns (e.g., cigarette), or concomitant bruising, FXs, or other trauma. Check for associated injuries (e.g., bruising, FXs)

HEADACHE

HX

- Onset, location, duration, severity, activity at time of onset
- Recent injury, possibility of concussion, sports
- HX of HA, change in severity or pattern, associated with menses F/C, N/V
- Recent viral illness, body aches, sinus problems, earache, sore throat, dental pain, facial pain
- Recent HA ("sentinel bleed"), HA worse with head position or Valsalva
- Visual changes, problems with hearing, speech, balance, ambulation
- Weakness of the extremities
- Confusion, weakness, lethargy, seizure
- Neck pain or stiffness
- Rash or lesions
- HA wakes pt from sleep, worse in the morning and improves throughout day
- Aura
- Drug use or withdrawal
- PMH or FH: migraines, metabolic or vascular DX
- Recent stressors, HX depression
- Meds
- Trauma

PE

- **General:** position of pt, level of distress, alert, lethargic
- **VS and SaO$_2$:** fever, tachycardia, pulse pressure
- **Skin:** PWD, moist, pale, rashes, or lesions
- **HEENT:**
  - **Head:** surface trauma, TTP, bony step-off, fontanels—if open
  - **Eyes:** sclera and conjunctiva, PERRLA, EOMI. Nystagmus, ptosis, diplopia. Periorbital STS, erythema, ecchymosis. Fundi: papilledema, hemorrhage. V/A
  - **Ears:** canals and TM clear. Battle's sign, hemotympanum, CSF leak
  - **Nose:** congestion, drainage. Nasal injury, septal hematoma, epistaxis, CSF rhinorrhea
  - **Face:** symmetry, strength, sensation, STS, trauma
  - **Mouth/Throat:** MMM, posterior pharynx clear; intraoral trauma, teeth, and mandible
- **Neck:** FROM without limitation or pain, NT to firm palp at midline; meningismus, lymphadenopathy
- **Chest:** NT, CTA
- **Heart:** RRR, no murmurs, rubs, or gallops; clear tones
- **Abd:** BS, NT
- **Back:** no spinal or CVAT
- **Extremities:** FROM, weakness, paresthesia, NT, distal CMS intact
- **Neuro:** A&O × 3, GCS 15, no focal neuro deficits. Speech, gait, Romberg, pronator drift

(cont.)

HEADACHE (cont.)

MDM/DDx

Many children present with headache related to benign viral illnesses or fever. The most common cause of acute recurrent HA in children is **migraine**. These classic throbbing HAs can be unilateral or bilateral and are associated with sensitivity to light and sound and can last hours to days. Pts may complain of fatigue, visual auras, hyperacusis, photophobia, and vomiting. In some cases of complicated migraine, the pt may experience focal or diffuse neurologic changes such as hemiplegia. **Tension HAs** are common and often associated with stress. They are usually fairly constant and do not cause N/V. Tension HA pain is usually at the base of the head and radiates to the neck; however, the neck is supple and nuchal rigidity is absent. Infections that cause headache, such as **meningitis** or **encephalitis**, usually are associated with fever and toxicity. Also consider **TMJ dysfunction** if there is pain, popping, or clicking of the joint. HAs that are worsening should prompt concern for intracranial etiology such as **subdural hematoma, intracranial bleed, tumor, abscess, AVM. Depression** and **situational stress** or **anxiety** are diagnoses of exclusion for pediatric HA.

MANAGEMENT

- Treatment generally directed toward supportive care (antiemetic and analgesia) followed by abortive and preventative management strategies
- **Labs:** usually not indicated
- **Imaging:** most children with HA and a normal exam do not require neuroimaging unless there is significant change in type or severity of usual headache pain. CT and/or MRI if new onset of severe HA, vomiting, seizures, or concern for structural etiology
- LP to R/O meningitis or after CT to R/O SAH. Infection: elevated opening pressure, elevated WBCs, and protein with low glucose
- **Meds:** Ibuprofen/acetaminophen; Toradol; steroids and DHE for intractable migraine, antiemetic
- **Migraine:** sumatriptan 10 mg nasal spray or injected, reserved for older adolescents; dihydroergotamine, contraindicated in complex migraine; prochlorperazine, may pretreat with Benadryl to prevent dystonic reaction
- **Other:** cluster HA may respond to 100% O_2 6 to 8 L/min via nonrebreather mask if started at onset of HA

(cont.)

HEADACHE (cont.)

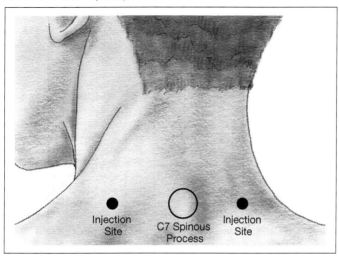

Lower paracervical intramuscular injection sites (for older adolescents)

LOWER PARACERVICAL INTRAMUSCULAR INJECTION

PROCEDURE NOTE: Procedure explained and consent obtained. Pt was placed in a seated position and the posterior seventh cervical vertebrae landmark palpated. Sterile drape and prep was done and injection sites were located 2 to 3 cm lateral to the spinous process. A 25 or 27 gauge needle was introduced 1 to 1.5 inches parallel to the top of the shoulder in a posterior to anterior direction. Bupivacaine 1.5 mL was slowly injected into the lower paraspinous muscle. The needle was withdrawn and the area massaged to promote absorption of the medication. DSD was applied. Lung sounds were CTA bilaterally after the procedure and the pt tolerated the procedure well. Pain level was ___/0 to 10 post procedure. Tolerated procedure well without complications

(cont.)

HEADACHE (cont.)
CRANIAL NERVES

I	Olfactory	Sense of smell
II	Optic	Visual acuity, visual fields, fundi
III	Oculomotor	Pupillary function, EOM function of IO, SR, MR, IR
IV	Trochlear	EOM function of SO
V	Trigeminal	Facial sensation to light touch, temperature, facial muscle strength, corneal reflex
VI	Abducens	EOM function of LR
VII	Facial	Symmetry of facial expressions (e.g., smile, frown, wrinkle forehead), taste anterior 2/3 of the tongue
VIII	Acoustic	Whisper test, tuning fork lateralization
IX	Glossopharyngeal	Gag reflex, swallow, taste posterior 1/3 of tongue
X	Vagus	Gag reflex, swallow, hoarseness, soft palate sensation
XI	Spinal accessory	Shoulder shrug and turn head against resistance
XII	Hypoglossal	Tongue symmetry, movement, strength

DICTATION/DOCUMENTATION

- **General:** WDWN, alert and active child in no acute distress. Not toxic appearing
- **VS and SaO$_2$:** afebrile
- **Skin:** PWD, normal texture and turgor
- **HEENT:**
  - **Head:** normocephalic, AT, fontanel normal
  - **Eyes:** V/A, visual fields normal. No ptosis or nystagmus. PERRLA, EOMI
  - **Ears:** no pre- or postauricular lymphadenopathy or erythema. Canals and TMs normal
  - **Nose:** no rhinorrhea or nasal flaring
  - **Face:** no asymmetry, normal strength, and sensation
  - **Mouth/Throat:** MMM, posterior pharynx clear
- **Neck:** supple, FROM, no meningismus, or lymphadenopathy
- **Chest:** no retractions, accessory muscle use. CTA. No wheezes, crackles, rhonchi
- **Heart:** RRR. No murmurs, rubs, or gallops.
- **Abd:** soft, BSA, NT, no distention, masses, hepatosplenomegaly
- **Back:** no spinal or CVAT
- **Extremities:** moves all extremities with good strength; neurovascular intact
- **Neuro:** A&O × 3, GCS 15, CN II–XII grossly intact. Motor and sensory exam nonfocal. Reflexes are symmetric. Speech is clear and gait is steady. Neg Romberg, no pronator drift

DON'T MISS!

- Occult head trauma
- Abusive head trauma in infants
- Acute confusion or AMS
- Fever and toxicity

HEAD INJURY

HX

- Time of injury, MOI (auto vs. pedestrian, ejection, significant fall, inflicted)
- Signs of concussion: headache (most frequent symptom), retrograde or anterograde amnesia, dizziness, tinnitus, mental fogginess, fatigue, irritability, observed and documented disorientation or confusion immediately after the event, impaired balance within 1 day after injury, slower reaction time within 2 days after injury, and impaired verbal learning and memory within 2 days after injury
- ALOC: gradual, sudden LOC, brief lucid interval
- HA, visual changes, seizure
- Blood/CSF leak nose/ears
- Neck/back pain, N/V (>twice)
- Distracting injury, suspected open or depressed skull FX
- Concern for basilar skull FX, depressed skull FX, or penetration of the skull (i.e., dog bite)
- Large scalp hematoma
- Fall (>5 ft for children >2 years of age or >3 ft for children <2 years of age)
- ALOC, disoriented, irritable, lethargic
- Serious MVC, unrestrained, auto versus pedestrian
- Wearing helmet
- Substance use (e.g., alcohol, IVDA, illicit drugs)
- PMH: risk of bleeding (e.g., hemophilia), VP shunt

PE

- **General:** WDWN, level of activity and interaction, distress. Strong cry, playful, withdrawn, irritable, lethargic
- **VS and SaO$_2$:** tachycardia or bradycardia significant for shock/neurogenic shock, pulse pressure
- **Skin:** PWD, texture, turgor, pallor, obvious surface trauma
- **HEENT:**
    - **Head:** normocephalic, fontanels (if open: anterior and posterior); ecchymosis, STS, bony step-off, deformity, nonfrontal hematoma
    - **Eyes:** periorbital ecchymosis, step-off; sclera and conjunctiva, PERRLA, EOMI
    - **Ears:** canals and TMs patent. Battle's sign, hemotympanum, CSF leak
    - **Nose:** STS, ecchymosis, deformity, epistaxis, CSF leak, septal hematoma; midfacial stability
    - **Face:** symmetry, surface trauma, strength, sensation
    - **Mouth/Throat:** intraoral trauma, teeth, and mandible
- **Neck:** FROM, NT to firm palp at midline
- **Chest:** NT, CTA; no wheezes, crackles, or rhonchi
- **Heart:** RRR; no murmurs, rubs, or gallops
- **Abd:** soft, BSA, nondistended, tenderness
- **Back:** spinal or CVA tenderness; flank ecchymosis
- **Pelvis:** NT to palpation and stable to compression, femoral pulses strong and equal
- **Extremities:** FROM, NT, strength and tone, neurovascular intact
- **Neuro:** alert, active, GCS 15, no focal neuro findings

(cont.)

HEAD INJURY (cont.)

MDM/DDx

The priority for evaluation of children with head trauma is to identify those pts with **minor head trauma** (e.g., abrasions, contusions, scalp hematomas) and those with **traumatic brain injury**. Children <2 years are more difficult to assess, may be asymptomatic despite having a TBI, and are at risk of **abusive head trauma**. A high index of suspicion must be maintained for abusive head trauma **(maltreatment)** and neuroimaging must be performed. Children >2 years with a normal neuro exam are felt to have minor head trauma if GCS of >14 at initial evaluation and there is no physical evidence of skull fracture. **Under 2 years:** suspicion of maltreatment, focal neuro deficit, scalp hematoma (occipital, parietal, or temporal), palpable skull FX, AMS, bulging fontanel, persistent vomiting, seizure, LOC >5 seconds, significant MOI; **over 2 years:** focal neuro deficit, palpable skull FX, seizure, AMS or prolonged LOC, significant MOI. **Concussion** is a trauma-induced TBI without structural injury and ranges from mild to severe. Persistent HA, confusion, and amnesia (retrograde and/or anterograde) with or without LOC are classic findings. Pts may also have HA, dizziness, lack of awareness of surroundings, N/V. A **mild TBI** is usually associated with LOC, disorientation, or vomiting, and GCS 13 to 15 (30 minutes after injury). **Moderate TBI** is present if GCS 9 to 12, whereas a GCS <8 indicates a **severe brain injury.**

MANAGEMENT

- **Mild injury with low risk:** analgesia, antiemetic, observation, very specific aftercare instructions and close F/U. Discharge criteria: observe 2 to 4 hours, no vomiting, normal neuro exam
- **Moderate risk:** may elect to observe closely 4 to 6 hours and CT for any worsening changes
- **Imaging:** noncontrast head CT indicated if:
    - **<2 Years:** suspicion of maltreatment, focal neuro deficit, scalp hematoma (occipital, parietal, or temporal), palpable skull FX, AMS, bulging fontanel, persistent vomiting, seizure, LOC >5 seconds, significant MOI
    - **>2 Years:** focal neuro deficit, palpable skull FX, seizure, AMS or prolonged LOC, significant MOI

(cont.)

HEAD INJURY (cont.)

DICTATION/DOCUMENTATION

- **General:** WDWN, alert, and active child in no acute distress
- **VS and SaO$_2$**
- **Skin:** PWD, no surface trauma
- **HEENT:**
  - **Head:** atraumatic, no palp deformity. Fontanel normal
  - **Eyes:** no periorbital STS, ecchymosis, step-off, deformity. Sclera and conjunctiva normal. PERRLA, EOMI
  - **Ears:** canals and TMs clear. No Battle's sign, hemotympanum, CSF leak
  - **Nose:** AT, NT, no epistaxis, CSF leak, septal hematoma. No midfacial instability
  - **Mouth/Throat:** no intraoral trauma, teeth and mandible stable, no malocclusion. Posterior pharynx clear
- **Neck:** no point tenderness, step-off, or deformity to firm palpation of the cervical spine at the midline. No spasm or paraspinal muscle tenderness. FROM without limitation or pain
- **Chest:** no surface trauma or asymmetry. NT without crepitus or deformity. Normal TV, no accessory muscle use. CTA bilaterally
- **Heart:** RRR. No murmurs, rubs, or gallops
- **Abd:** flat, no surface trauma or distention. BSA. Soft, nontender to palpation, no guarding, rebound, or masses. Good femoral pulses
- **Back:** no contusions, ecchymosis, or abrasions noted. NT without step-off or deformity to firm palpation of the thoracic and lumbar spine.
- **Pelvis:** NT to palpation and stable to compression
- **GU:** normal external genitalia with no blood at the meatus (if applicable)
- **Rectal:** normal tone
- **Extremities:** no surface trauma. AT, NT. FROM. Distal motor, neurovascular supply intact
- **Neuro:** A&O ×4, GCS 15, CN II–XII grossly intact. Motor and sensory exam nonfocal. Reflexes are symmetric. Speech is clear and gait is steady

● TIPS

- Scalp hematoma <2 years associated with increased risk of skull FX or intracranial bleed
- Significant MOI: auto versus child or bike riding without helmet, fall >3 ft, struck in the head by heavy or high-impact object
- Children may have significant brain injury with absent clues such as vomiting, change in behavior, or complaint of HA
- Listen to caregiver concerns that child is "acting different or funny"

DON'T MISS!

- Maltreatment
- Cervical trauma
- Facial trauma

EYE PAIN

HX

- Onset, duration, unilateral, or bilateral
- Redness, discharge, tearing, itching, burning, swelling, ptosis or proptosis, FB sensation
- Restricted or painful eye movement
- Visual changes: photophobia, diplopia, decreased or loss of vision, flashes of light
- Trauma: blunt or penetrating
- Chemical exposure
- Nasal congestion, cough, fever, ear pain, rash, joint swelling
- Facial lesions, redness, swelling
- Baseline vision, previous HA or eye problems, surgeries. Corrective glasses, contacts, or protective eyewear
- Exposed to an ill contact
- Maternal history of STIs (neonates)
- Past medical history: HA, DM, CA, JIA, herpes
- Allergies

PE

- **General:** WDWN, level of activity and interaction, distress. Strong cry, playful, withdrawn, irritable, lethargic
- **VS and SaO$_2$:** afebrile
- **Skin:** PWD, texture, turgor
- **HEENT:**
    - **Head:** normocephalic, fontanels (anterior and posterior)
    - **Eyes:** V/A; periorbital STS, erythema, warmth. Lid margins and eversion: No FB, lesion, inflammation. Lashes equally distributed; note nits or lice. EOMI or tracking: note restricted or painful. Sclera and conjunctiva: note erythema, inflammation, crusting, or discharge. VF: full to confrontation (use a brightly colored toy, object, or pen light for a younger child, the standard method for an older child). PERRLA, red-light reflex symmetrical in size, color, and clarity. Fundi: optic disk
    - **Ears:** pain on manipulation of tragus. Pre- or postauricular lymphadenopathy, tenderness, or erythema over mastoid. Canals patent without erythema, edema, discharge, cerumen, FB. TMs pearly grey with good light reflex; effusion, fluid level, bullae
    - **Nose:** mucosa pink and patent, rhinorrhea or nasal flaring. Herpetic lesion on tip of nose
    - **Mouth/Throat:** MMM, strawberry tongue, intraoral vesicles, ulcerations, palatal petechiae. Drooling or stridor. Posterior pharynx clear without lesions, erythema, exudates, or asymmetry
- **Neck:** supple, FROM, meningismus, lymphadenopathy
- **Chest:** retractions, accessory muscle use, grunting, stridor. CTA; no wheezes, crackles, or rhonchi
- **Heart:** RRR, no murmurs, rubs, or gallops
- **Abd:** soft, BSA, nondistended; no tenderness, masses, hepatosplenomegaly
- **GU:** normal external genitalia; no lesion, rash, erythema
- **Back:** spinal or CVAT
- **Extremities:** FROM, strength and tone, neurovascularly intact
- **Neuro:** alert, active, GCS 15, no focal neuro findings

(cont.)

EYE PAIN (cont.)

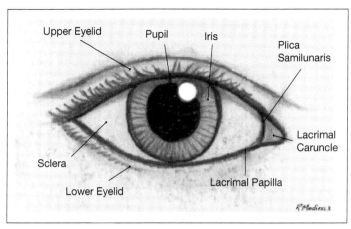

Anatomy of the external eye

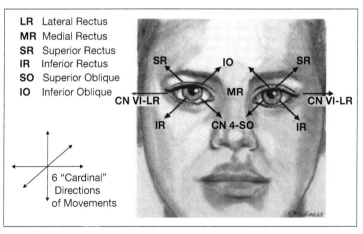

Extraocular movements

(cont.)

EYE PAIN (cont.)

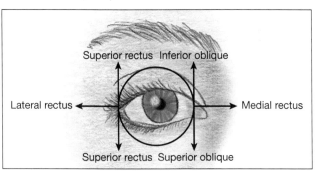

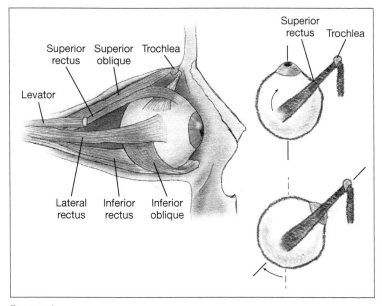

Eye muscles

(cont.)

EYE PAIN (cont.)

MDM/DDx

Common causes of red eye include infection, trauma, chemical exposure, and allergic or inflammatory conditions. **Conjunctivitis** may be caused by a virus, herpes, bacteria, or allergy. Itching, watery discharge, and a mild amount of mucus, often associated with a URI and an ipsilateral preauricular bilateral node is consistent with **viral conjunctivitis**. Also itchy, **allergic conjunctivitis** causes watery eyes associated with other allergic symptoms. **Bacterial conjunctivitis** more often has thick mucoid discharge and matting of the eyelids, usually without associated URI symptoms. **Herpetic conjunctivitis** is a sight-threatening disorder, characterized by a dendritic appearance on fluorescein stain, or Hutchinson's sign (vesicular lesions of the nose). **Iritis** affects the deeper structures of the eye and presents with unilateral direct photophobia, consensual photophobia pain, and tearing, without mucoid or purulent discharge. **Preseptal/periorbital cellulitis** causes periorbital pain, erythema, edema, and induration, and should be monitored closely for extension of infection into deeper ocular structures leading to **orbital cellulitis. Corneal abrasions** are a common cause of a painful red eye and are associated with photophobia, tearing, and decreased vision. A **corneal ulcer** is an uncommon but very serious infection that is sometimes a complication to an abrasion. It appears as an opacified area of the cornea and requires prompt treatment to prevent corneal perforation or permanent loss of vision. Blood in the anterior chamber, or **hyphema**, may be visible on exam or seen on SLE. Hyphema causes pain, decreased V/A, and photophobia. **Orbital rim FXs** following trauma cause pain, periorbital bony step-off or deformity, ecchymosis, subconjunctival hemorrhage, decreased or limited EOM, and possible palpable subcutaneous air. **Chemical burns** are painful and are associated with significant tearing, redness, possible opacification, and decreased V/A. Determination of acid/base imbalance by pH measurement is essential to guide management

MANAGEMENT

- **Labs:** CBC with differential, CRP, ESR, chem panel, blood culture with signs of systemic infectious or inflammatory illness; full septic workup for neonates with suspected gonococcal infection, including conjunctiva swab for Gram stain, viral, and bacterial culture. NAAT is more sensitive than culture for GC and chlamydia
- **Imaging:** CT scan of the orbits with IV contrast for trauma or periorbital cellulitis

(cont.)

EYE PAIN (cont.)

MEDICAL

- **Allergic:** supportive care, artificial tears, cool compresses, Naphcon A 1 to 2 gtts QID
- **Conjunctivitis: viral:** supportive care, artificial tears, and cool compresses or ocular antihistamine/mast cell stabilizer of choice
- **Conjunctivitis: bacterial:** trimethoprim/polymyxin B (Polytrim) 1 to 2 gtts QID ×1 week, aminoglycosides (gentamicin, tobramycin, erythromycin) 0.5-inch ribbon QID for 1 week
- **Gonococcal:** ceftriaxone 1 g IM, infants 50 mg/kg/IV (max 125 mg)
- **Chlamydial:** erythromycin ophthalmic ointment and oral erythromycin 50 mg/kg/d divided QID for 14 days in neonate
- **Herpetic:** ophthalmology consult; trifluridine drops 1 gtt q4h for 7 to 14 days; acyclovir IV or PO may also be used
- **Preseptal cellulitis:** ceftriaxone 50 mg/kg × 1 dose followed by augmentin 50 mg/kg/d of amoxicillin PO divided BID × 10 days; an alternative alone or in combination may be TMP/SMX 8 to 12 mg/kg/d divided PO BID or clindamycin 10 mg/kg/d PO TID to cover MRSA
- **Periorbital cellulitis:** ophthalmology consult; broad spectrum IV antibiotics (vancomycin 10–15 mg/kg BID or clindamycin 10 mg/kg TID and ceftriaxone 100 mg/kg divided BID)

TRAUMA

- **Corneal FB:** topical anesthesia, tetanus status, removal with moistened cotton tip applicator, eye spud, sterile needle
- **Corneal abrasion:** trimethoprim/polymyxin B (Polytrim) 1 to 2 gtts QID for 1 week, aminoglycosides (gentamicin, tobramycin, erythromycin) 0.5-inch ribbon QID for 1 week, ibuprofen (10 mg/kg/dose q8h or acetaminophen 15 mg/kg/dose q6h)
- **Hyphema:** ophthalmology consult; cycloplegics for comfort (atropine gtts <1 year old 0.25% 1 gtt TID; 1 to 5 years old 0.5% 1 gtt TID; >5 years old 1% 1 gtt TID)
- **Orbital fracture:** ophthalmology consult, urgent repair with entrapment of extraocular muscles, antibiotics to prevent secondary infection (cephalexin 50 mg/kg TID or TMP/SMX 8–12 mg/kg/d divided PO BID × 10 days)
- **Chemical burns:** verify whether agent is alkali or acid, check pH in the palpebral space, immediate and continuous irrigation until the pH is neutralized by pH paper (7.4), recheck pH 20 minutes after discontinuing irrigation, topical antibiotics to prevent secondary infection

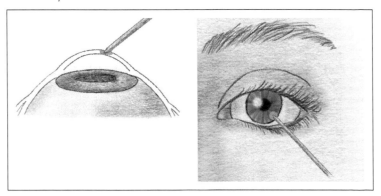

Superficial corneal foreign body removal

(cont.)

EYE PAIN (cont.)

DICTATION/DOCUMENTATION

- **General:** WDWN, alert and active child in no acute distress. Not toxic appearing
- **VS and SaO$_2$:** afebrile
- **Skin:** PWD, normal texture and turgor
- **HEENT:**
  - **Head:** normocephalic, fontanel normal
  - **Eyes:** V/A, no periorbital STS, erythema, warmth, induration. Lids and lashes clear without erythema, inflammation, crusting, or discharge (and note if still open). No nits/lice. Lids everted and no evidence of FB, lesion, inflammation. EOMI or tracks normally without limitation or complaint of pain. VF FROM. Sclera and conjunctivae normal, no erythema, cobblestone, lesion, drainage, PERRLA; red-light reflex symmetrical in size, color, and clarity
  - **Ears:** no pre- or postauricular lymphadenopathy or erythema. Canals and TMs normal
  - **Nose:** no rhinorrhea or nasal flaring, no lesions on tip of nose
  - **Mouth/Throat:** lips moist, MMM, no intraoral lesions, no drooling or stridor. No asymmetry of posterior pharynx, uvula midline, no erythema or exudates
- **Neck:** supple, FROM, no meningismus or lymphadenopathy
- **Chest:** no retractions, accessory muscle use, grunting, stridor. CTA. No wheezes, crackles, rhonchi
- **Heart:** RRR, no murmurs, rubs, or gallops
- **Abd:** soft, BSA, NT, no distention or masses, no HSM
- **GU:** normal external genitalia, no rash or lesions
- **Back:** no spinal or CVAT
- **Extremities:** FROM, strength and tone, neurovascularly intact
- **Neuro:** alert, active, GCS 15, no focal neuro findings

EYE PROCEDURE NOTE

Topical anesthetic was instilled with good anesthesia using _____ (e.g., proparacaine). Fluorescein stain of the R/L eye was performed without uptake of dye. No epithelial defect was noted. No foreign body, ulcer, or dendritic lesions. Upper lid was everted and no foreign body or lesions were noted. Slit lamp exam was performed. No fluorescein uptake or epithelial defect noted. Anterior chamber is clear without cell or flare. No Seidel sign. Normal saline irrigation/eye wash solution was performed and the pt tolerated the procedure well, with no adverse reactions or complications. Note intraocular pressure readings with tonometer (normal eye pressure range 10–20 mmHg)

(cont.)

EYE PAIN (cont.)

⊙ TIPS

- Good relief of pain with ophthalmic anesthesia is reassuring; for deeper structure involvement pain will not improve even with the use of ophthalmic eye drops
- V/A: 20/40 normal
- Use symbols for verbal but preliterate child of 4 to 6 years (e.g., Snellen Tumbling E test)
- 20/20 >6 years of age Snellen chart

DON'T MISS!

- Corneal epithelial defects—fluorescein stain all cases of red eye
- Herpetic conjunctivitis
- Corneal ulcerations
- Any child with eye trauma should be evaluated for maltreatment
- Pediatric ophthalmology consult for suspected child maltreatment to evaluate for retinal hemorrhages associated with abusive head trauma

EARACHE

HX

- Onset, duration
- F/C, N/V/D, posttussive emesis, irritability, loss of appetite
- Eye drainage, runny nose, congestion, sinus pain
- Ear pain, pulling at ears, drainage, bleeding, foul odor, itching, feeling of fullness
- Cough, sputum production
- Headache, ringing in ears, hearing loss, dizziness, trouble with balance
- Local trauma, exposure to water, foreign objects, day care
- Recent altitude changes, head injury
- Poor feeding or behavior changes in children
- Immunosuppressed, DM, HIV, atopic dermatitis, psoriasis, seborrheic dermatitis
- Smoke exposure, environmental irritants, travel, sick contacts
- FB ear/nose
- Trauma
- HX: prematurity, previous episodes
- Immunizations, medications

PE

- **General:** alert, in no acute distress, no ataxia
- **VS and SaO$_2$:** fever, tachycardia, tachypnea
- **Skin:** PWD, normal texture and turgor; lesions, rash
- **HEENT:**
  - **Head:** NT, normocephalic, normal fontanel (if still open)
  - **Eyes:** PERRLA, EOMI, sclera and conjunctiva clear, drainage/discharge, edema, allergic shiners, periorbital STS or erythema, nystagmus
  - **Ears:** pre- or postauricular lymphadenopathy, erythema, or lesions. Swelling, erythema, or pain on movement of tragus or auricle; protrusion of auricle. Canal: erythema, edema, exudate, cerumen, FB TM: erythema, bulging, retraction, landmarks, fluid level, bullae, perforation, cerumen, mobility of TM with insufflation (cerumen removal for adequate exam if needed)
  - **Nose:** rhinorrhea, flare, hyperemic, snoring, boggy, hyperemic, sinuses TTP/erythema
  - **Mouth/Throat:** MMM, posterior pharynx clear, no erythema, exudate, vesicles, petechiae, halitosis, erythema, exudate, stridor, drooling
- **Neck:** supple, NT, FROM, no meningismus, or lymphadenopathy
- **Chest:** CTA, no wheezes, rhonchi, crackles; retractions, O$_2$ sat
- **Heart:** RRR, no murmurs, rubs, or gallops
- **Abd:** soft, NT, BSA, no HSM
- **Back:** spinal or CVAT
- **Extremities:** FROM
- **Neuro:** A&O ×3, GCS 15, no focal neuro deficits, normal behavior for age

(cont.)

EARACHE (cont.)

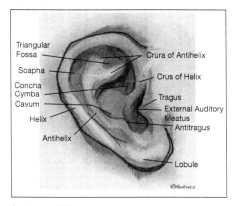

Anatomy of the ear

MDM/DDx

Evaluation of **ear pain (otalgia)** is directed toward determining whether the origin of pain is from the ear or referred from surrounding structures. Ear pain can be caused by acute AOE, AOM, serous otitis, perforated TM, or infection of the outer ear. FBs, local trauma, or cerumen impaction can also cause ear pain. **AOE** is often caused by exposure to water or local trauma such as Q-tip use. Often caused by staph or strep but considered fungal if recent Abx use. Pain associated with OME can be severe. **Malignant otitis externa** is a potentially life-threatening condition that is often caused by fungal infection; more common in diabetics or the immunosuppressed. **AOM** incidence peaks in younger children 6 to 24 months and is often caused by *S. pneumo* or *H. flu*. AOM associated with hearing loss, tinnitus, vertigo, and pain may indicate the presence of effusion and limited TM mobility. Drainage from the ear canal should prompt consideration of **ruptured TM**. Prolonged episodes of otalgia with pain deep inside or behind the ear may indicate **acute mastoiditis**, a less common but serious infection of the temporal bone associated with hearing loss and other complications. All pts with otitis media should be evaluated for **pneumonia, dehydration**, or **sepsis**. Dental or **intraoral infections** or **TMJ dysfunction** can present as acute ear pain

(cont.)

EARACHE (cont.)

MANAGEMENT

- Initial treatment of otalgia of any etiology is adequate **analgesia**; Tylenol or ibuprofen; topical anesthetic: antipyrine/benzocaine gtts if TM intact
- AOE: cerumen removal if indicated, acetic acid. Keep canal clean and dry. Possible CT/MRI if severe
    - **Meds:** polymyxin B/neomycin/hydrocortisone 4 gtts QID × 7 d (use suspension not solution in case of perforation); ofloxacin 0.3% sol 5 gtts BID × 7 d; ciprofloxacin/hydrocortisone 3 gtts BID (not for perforation)
- AOM: most cases of pediatric AOM improve spontaneously and Abx are not indicated
    - **"Wait and see"** approach for well children 6 to 24 months (or older) with mild to moderate unilateral ear pain. Provide Abx, clear instructions for supportive care, potential complications, and ensure close follow-up; start Abx if not better in 2 to 3 days. Need parental involvement in treatment options
- **Abx indicated:** >6 months with severe unilateral or bilateral ear pain for over 48 hours and temp >102° Fahrenheit; older child who is toxic appearing, failed treatment, immunosuppressed, comorbidities
    - **Meds:** amoxicillin is first-line Abx (unless failed Abx in the last month) 45 mg/kg BID × 5 to 7 days; amoxicillin/clavulanate 45 mg/kg BID if no improvement in 3 days or worsening SXS; azithromycin if pen allergic; ceftriaxone if toxic or unable to tolerate POs
- **Mastoiditis:** possible CT/MRI, admission, ENT consultation
    - **Meds:** vancomycin 40 mg/kg/d divided Q6 h; ceftriaxone 50 mg/kg IV daily (>12 years use 1 g/d); clindamycin 7.5 mg/kg IV QID

DICTATION/DOCUMENTATION

- **General:** awake and alert, not toxic appearing
- **VS and SaO$_2$**
- **Skin:** PWD
- **HEENT:**
    - **Head:** normocephalic, NT
    - **Eyes:** sclera and conjunctiva clear, PERRLA, EOMI
    - **Ears:** no pre- or postauricular lymphadenopathy or erythema; canals are clear, no erythema, edema, exudates. No cerumen impaction. TMs normal or bulging or retraction. Good light reflex or dull. No fluid level, vesicles, or bullae. No perforation
    - **Nose/Face:** no rhinorrhea, congestion, nasal flaring, bleeding, no foul odor/discharge, frontal or maxillary sinus TTP
    - **Mouth/Throat:** MMM, posterior pharynx clear, no erythema or exudate
- **Neck:** supple, FROM, NT, no lymphadenopathy, no meningismus
- **Chest:** CTA
- **Abd:** soft, BSA, NT
- **Extremities:** FROM, no swelling, edema, tenderness
- **Neuro:** A&O ×3, GCS 15, no focal neuro deficits, normal behavior for age

(cont.)

EARACHE (cont.)

CERUMEN REMOVAL PROCEDURE NOTE

Procedure explained and consent obtained. Cerumen was removed from the L/R ear canal with a loop in order to visualize the tympanic membrane. Tolerated procedure well with no complications

DON'T MISS!

- Toxic appearing or unable to tolerate oral fluids
- Complications: meningismus, mastoiditis, pneumonia
- Ear FB

FOREIGN BODIES: EAR/NOSE

HX

- Onset
- Location—ask about all orifices
- Duration
- Characteristics: type of FB, assoc signs and SXS (e.g., object can be visualized, nasal drainage or congestion, coughing/choking), verbal admission by child/witnessed by caregiver, parent may have attempted to remove, at home remedies
- Local pain, edema, erythema, signs of infection
- Bleeding, D/C, unilateral foul smell from ear/nostril
- N/V, nystagmus, vertigo, ataxia

PE

- **General:** WDWN, level of activity and interaction, distress
- **VS and SaO$_2$:** afebrile
- **Skin:** PWD, texture, turgor
- **HEENT:**
    - **Head:** normocephalic, AT
    - **Eyes:** PERRLA, EOMI, sclera, and conjunctiva
    - **Ears:** pain on palpation of tragus. Drainage, blood, odor at external auditory meatus. Canals: erythema, edema, blood, discharge, FB. TMs: normal, occluded, perforation
    - **Nose:** mucosa pink and patent, epistaxis, discharge, edema, foul odor, FB, septum
    - **Mouth/Throat:** MMM, posterior pharynx, FB, drooling, stridor
- **Neck:** supple, FROM
- **Chest:** retractions, accessory muscle use, lungs clear to auscultation; wheezes, rales, or rhonchi
- **Heart:** RRR
- **Abd:** BSA, soft, NT

MDM/DDx

Symptoms and course depend on the type of FB. **Alkaline batteries (e.g., button batteries) cause alkaline** burns and liquefaction necrosis, and must be removed urgently. **Insect FBs** cause pain by movement or stinging, causing a local inflammatory response or anaphylaxis. **Ear FBs** that penetrate the TM have potential for middle/inner ear damage and require immediate attention (e.g., Q-tips, pencil tips, hair pins). Delayed discovery of FB can lead to inflammation and infection

MANAGEMENT

- **Labs:** generally not indicated. Septic workup if toxic appearing
- **Imaging:** temporal bone CT if unable to visualize foreign body or liquefaction necrosis is suspected (ear). Plain nasal films for button batteries or magnets suspected and not able to visualize.

(cont.)

FOREIGN BODIES: EAR/NOSE (cont.)

FB REMOVAL—EAR

- **Irrigation** may be adequate for small inorganic objects or insects (instill mineral oil or 1% lidocaine into canal to kill insect prior to irrigation). Irrigation contraindicated with TM tubes, perforation of the TM, removal of vegetable matter (e.g., beans), or button batteries
- **Instrumentation** under direct visualization requires good restraint, lighting, and possible sedation. Place child in supine position with the affected ear up. Use alligator or bayonet forceps to remove soft objects, irregular edges, or insects. Round or breakable objects are more easily removed with blunt right-angle hook, angled wire loop, or angled flexible cerumen curette. Freely mobile spherical objects are best removed with suction

FB REMOVAL—NOSE

- **Positive pressure technique:** occlude child's unaffected nostril with direct pressure and have the parent blow mouth to mouth by firmly sealing his or her mouth over the child's, giving a short, sharp puff of air into the child's mouth. A bag-valve mask may also be used for positive pressure
- **Instrumentation:** under direct visualization requires good restraint, lighting, and possible sedation
- **Position:** child in supine position with head immobilized. Instill topical vasoconstrictor (0.5% phenylephrine spray) into affected nostril and 1% lidocaine without epinephrine drops for local anesthesia (up to 5 mg/kg) 5 minutes before procedure. Insert nasal speculum for direct visualization. Use alligator forceps or nasal forceps to remove nonocclusive compressible objects. Round or breakable objects can be removed with a blunt right-angle hook, angled wire loop, or otorhino balloon FB extractor advanced beyond the object and withdrawn
- **FB removal nose/ear—"super glue" technique** (cyanoacrylate glue): apply a small amount of glue to a cotton swab, press onto visualized object for 60 seconds and then remove FB

DICTATION/DOCUMENTATION

- **General:** WDWN, alert, and active child in no acute distress
- **VS and SaO$_2$**
- **Skin:** PWD, normal texture and turgor
- **HEENT:**
  - **Head:** normocephalic, fontanel normal
  - **Eyes:** PERRLA, EOMI, sclera and conjunctiva normal
  - **Ears:** FB (describe) noted in canal; swelling, erythema, drainage, blood. TM intact without perforation
  - **Nose:** no rhinorrhea or epistaxis. FB (describe) noted in nostril
  - **Mouth/Throat:** MMM, posterior pharynx clear, no drooling or stridor
- **Neck:** supple, FROM
- **Chest:** respirations unlabored, CTA. No wheezes, crackles, rhonchi
- **Heart:** RRR
- **Abd:** soft, BSA, NT

(cont.)

FOREIGN BODIES: EAR/NOSE (cont.)

NOSE/EAR PROCEDURE FB REMOVAL NOTE

Procedure explained and consent obtained. Child restrained and placed supine. FB (describe) was visualized in external auditory canal/nostril. Note technique used for removal and number of attempts; however, discontinue attempts if significant bleeding. FB was expelled/removed intact. Canal/nostril reexamined and no other FBs were visualized in canals/nares. No TM perforation. No bleeding. Tolerated procedure well with no complications

DON'T MISS!

- Urgent ENT consultation: unable to remove button batteries or paired magnets, glass, impacted items, or penetrating FBs

- Always examine both ears and both nostrils for additional FB. Remember to reexamine after removal for patency/complete FB removal

FACIAL PAIN/INJURY

HX
- Pain, tingling, or motor/sensation changes
- Trauma: MOI: play, sports, traffic accidents, assault, child maltreatment, time of injury
- LOC, visual problems, neck pain, vomiting
- Concomitant trauma
- PMH
- SH: consider maltreatment
- Tetanus immunization HX
- Allergies

PE
- **General:** WDWN, level of activity and interaction, distress
- **VS and SaO$_2$**
- **Skin:** PWD, surface trauma
- **HEENT:**
  - **Head:** normocephalic, atraumatic, surface trauma, fontanels (anterior and posterior) flat, full, or bulging
  - **Eyes:** V/A. Periorbital STS, ecchymosis, crepitus, TTP. Sclera and conjunctivae clear; subconjunctival hemorrhage. PERRLA, EOMI, or tracks normally
  - **Ears:** (Ramsay Hunt—rare in children) hearing loss affected ear. Surface trauma of external ear; blood or CSF in canal, TM perforation, hemotympanum, Battle's sign
  - **Nose:** surface trauma, deformity, epistaxis, CSF lead, septal hematoma
  - **Face:** (Bell's palsy/Ramsay Hunt—rare in children) unilateral facial paralysis, tingling/numbness of the cheek/mouth
  - **Mouth/Throat:** surface trauma of lips; laceration involving vermillion border. Injury of frenulum, tongue, gingiva, intraoral STS, ecchymosis, abrasion, lacerations (note whether laceration crosses vermillion border). Teeth and mandible stable; malocclusion; trismus. Posterior pharynx clear. Normal occlusive ability using tongue depressor. TMJ, NT
- **Neck:** surface trauma, spasm, mass. FROM. Midline TTP, step-off, deformity of posterior cervical spine
- **Chest:** NP, asymmetry, CTA
- **Heart:** RRR
- **Abd:** surface trauma, soft, BSA, NT
- **Back:** surface trauma, spinal tenderness
- **Extremities:** AT, NT, FROM
- **Neuro:** alert, active, GCS 15, no focal neurological findings, normal behavior for age

(cont.)

FACIAL PAIN/INJURY (cont.)

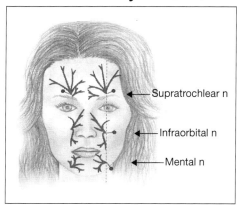

Supratrochlear n

Infraorbital n

Mental n

Location of the facial nerves

MDM/DDx

FACE PAIN

Bell's palsy: unilateral facial nerve paralysis may occur in the pediatric population

Ramsay Hunt syndrome (herpes zoster oticus): Rare complication of HZV can cause unilateral facial paralysis and hearing loss in the affected ear

FACIAL TRAUMA

Carefully evaluate all facial injuries for concomitant head and neck injuries, and airway patency. Suspect child **maltreatment** if there are inconsistencies in history, MOI, developmental level of child, or unexplained injuries. **Facial FXs** are uncommon in children <10 years old; large head protects smaller facial structures. **Orbital FXs** may be associated with local anesthesia, diplopia, limited upward gaze, enophthalmos. **Anterior basilar skull FXs** are frequently associated with periorbital ecchymosis "raccoon eyes" and CSF rhinorrhea. Malocclusion is commonly found with **mandible and/or maxillary FXs.** Instability of the palate suggests a **LeFort FX.** Eyelid injuries that involve the medial canthus can be associated with nasolacrimal duct injuries. **Deep lacerations** of the face require careful evaluation for injury to facial nerves, muscles, and parotid and salivary glands. Evaluate all **lip lacerations** for disruption of the vermillion border, which affects cosmetic outcome. **Frenulum lacerations** may be associated with child maltreatment (forced feeding)

MANAGEMENT

FACIAL PAIN

- **Bell's palsy:** Protect affected eye (artificial tears, tape eye shut at night). Consider prednisone if onset of symptoms <72 hours (use with caution if immunosuppressed, DM, pregnant, infection, liver/renal disease, PUD). Possible antivirals in conjunction with corticosteroids if viral etiology suspected: acyclovir or valacyclovir
- **Ramsay Hunt syndrome:** Use acyclovir and high dose steroids

FACIAL TRAUMA

- **ABCs,** control bleeding, ice, analgesia (see "Pain"). Elevate HOB if C-spine cleared

(cont.)

FACIAL PAIN/INJURY (cont.)

IMAGING

- Nasal x-rays of the nose for suspected FX are not indicated as nasal structures are largely cartilage and poorly visualized; nasal films expose child to significant radiation of the head and brain
- Facial x-rays are difficult to interpret in children and facial/orbital CT is preferred. Panorex is preferred imaging for FXs of maxilla or mandible
- Noncontrast head CT for suspected skull FX or intracranial injury or abusive head trauma

CSF LEAK

- Confirm by placing a drop of drainage from nose or ear on filter paper. Darker blood is surrounded by serum and yellowish CSF appearing as a "target/halo/ring" sign. CSF will also test positive for glucose by dipstick

MEDS

- Tetanus prophylaxis
- Prophylactic Abx may not be warranted although ophthalmology and ENT specialists frequently advise prophylactic Abx for orbital fractures
- Prophylactic Abx (5-day course) for animal/human bite, deep intraoral lacerations involving nasal cartilage, extensive contamination

DICTATION/DOCUMENTATION

- **General:** WDWN, alert, and active child in no acute distress
- **VS and SaO$_2$**
- **Skin:** PWD, no ecchymosis, abrasion, lacerations
- **HEENT:**
  - **Head:** AT, NT, fontanels normal without bulging
  - **Eyes:** V/A, no periorbital STS, ecchymosis, TTP. EOMI or tracks normally without limitation or complaint of pain; symmetrical upward gaze. V/F FROM
  - Sclera and conjunctivae normal, no subconjunctival hemorrhage; corneas grossly clear. PERRLA, red-light reflex symmetrical in size, color, and clarity
  - **Ears:** no surface trauma of outer ear. No CSF or blood in canal, no TM perforation or hemotympanum, Battle's sign
  - **Mouth/Throat:** no periorbital trauma, no intraoral trauma, teeth and mandible stable; no malocclusion or trismus
- **Neck:** no point tenderness, step-off, or deformity to firm palpation of the posterior cervical spine at the midline; no spasm or mass, FROM without limitation or complaint of pain
- **Chest:** no surface trauma, no TTP. CTA. No wheezes, crackles, rhonchi
- **Heart:** RRR
- **Abd:** BSA, no surface trauma, no TTP, no guarding or rigidity
- **Back:** no surface trauma, no spinal or CVAT
- **Extremities:** AT, no TTP, moves all extrems with good strength, distal neurovascular intact
- **Neuro:** alert, active, GCS 15, cranial nerves II–XII intact, no focal neurological findings

(cont.)

FACIAL PAIN/INJURY (cont.)

⊃TIPS

- **Facial wound repair** (see also "Wound")
- First suture carefully placed at lip margin to approximate lacerations crossing the vermillion border to ensure optimal cosmetic outcome
- Frenulum lacerations rarely require surgical repair
- Tongue lacerations should be closed: >1 cm and extend into the muscle layer, deep lacerations on the lateral border, large flaps or gaps in the tongue, likely to cause dysfunction (anterior split tongue)

DON'T MISS!

- Concomitant intracranial or cervical spine injuries
- Possibility of child maltreatment (e.g., abusive head trauma)
- Nasal septal hematoma (necrosis and erosion of the septum can result)

THROAT PAIN

HX

- Onset, duration, severity
- Painful swallowing and/or speaking, drooling, muffled voice
- Pain with movement of neck, torticollis
- Fever, N/V/D, cough
- Rash
- Preceding URI symptoms
- Trauma, chemical exposure
- Immunization history

PE

- **General:** WDWN, level of activity and interaction, distress. Strong cry
- **VS:** afebrile
- **Skin:** PWD, normal texture and turgor, no cyanosis or pallor, rash (scarlatiniform, viral exanthem)
- **HEENT:**
  - **Head:** normocephalic without evidence of trauma. Fontanel (anterior and posterior) flat, full, or bulging; mastoid tenderness or discoloration
  - **Eyes:** sclera white and conjunctivae pink. PERRLA, EOMI
  - **Ears:** no pain on palpation of tragus. Canals patent without erythema, edema, discharge, or foreign body. TMs pearly grey with good light reflex. No effusion. No pre- or postauricular lymphadenopathy
  - **Nose:** mucosa pink and patent, without rhinorrhea or nasal flaring
  - **Mouth/Throat:** no drooling or stridor. MMM, no strawberry tongue. No vesicles, petechiae, ulcerations, or inflammation. No asymmetry or bulging of posterior soft palate. Uvula midline without edema or erythema. Posterior pharynx clear without lesions, erythema, exudates, or asymmetry. No pain on palpation of jaw or TMJ. No evidence of trauma or foreign body

Centor Criteria

C—Cough absent, or the incorrect but memorable "Can't Cough"
E—Exudate
N—Nodes
T—Temperature elevated
OR—Young OR old modifier (<15 or >45 years of age)
Use only in patients with recent onset (≤3 days) acute pharyngitis

- **Neck:** supple, FROM, no meningismus, torticollis, or lymphadenopathy
- **Chest:** no retractions, no grunting, or stridor. CTA; no wheezes, crackles, or rhonchi
- **Heart:** RRR, no murmurs, rubs, or gallops
- **Abd:** soft, BSA, nondistended, NT, no HSM
- **Back:** no spinal or CVAT
- **Extremities:** FROM, good strength and tone bilaterally. Neurovascularly intact.
- **Neuro:** alert, active, with age appropriate behavior, GCS 15, no focal neurological findings noted

(cont.)

THROAT PAIN (cont.)

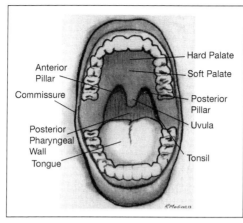

Anatomy of the mouth and throat

Labels in figure: Anterior Pillar, Commissure, Posterior Pharyngeal Wall, Tongue, Hard Palate, Soft Palate, Posterior Pillar, Uvula, Tonsil

MDM/DDx

The most common cause of sore throat is **viral pharyngitis**, followed by **group A beta-hemolytic streptococcus**. **Strep pharyngitis** typically includes fever, pharyngeal exudate, palatal petechiae, and anterior cervical adenopathy. Noninfectious causes of sore throat include chemical/environmental irritation, FB, and trauma (e.g., penetrating injuries to the posterior pharynx). Unimmunized children are at risk for epiglottis and diphtheria. Life-threatening complications (caused by airway compromise) of acute pharyngitis can lead to **deep neck infections: peritonsillar abscess/cellulitis:** unilateral tonsillar/peritonsillar swelling, uvular deviation, trismus, and muffled voice; **retropharyngeal abscess:** neck pain, neck mass, decreased ROM of neck (particularly extension), unilateral posterior pharyngeal bulge, usually occurs in children less than 4 years old; **parapharyngeal abscess:** swelling of the parotid area, trismus, and tonsillar prolapse; **epiglottitis:** toxic appearance, high fever, stridor, and drooling; **diphtheria:** thick pharyngeal membrane and marked cervical adenopathy. Systemic inflammatory conditions include **Kawasaki disease:** fever, mucositis, conjunctivitis, peripheral erythema, truncal rash, cervical adenopathy; **Stevens–Johnson syndrome:** vesicular and ulcerative lesions of the mucosa, and diffuse rash; and **Lemierre syndrome:** rare, severe pharyngitis, jugular venous thrombophlebitis, and dissemination by septic emboli. **Gonococcal pharyngitis** should be considered in children/adolescents who are sexually active or those with suspected sexual abuse

(cont.)

THROAT PAIN (cont.)

MANAGEMENT

LABS
- Rapid strep test (70%–90% sensitive) and/or culture for suspected strep pharyngitis. Monospot for children who have been symptomatic for >7 days. CBC with diff, ESR, CRP, and blood culture if infection is suspected and child is ill appearing

IMAGING
- Soft tissue lateral neck x-ray in children who are ill appearing, have significant difficulty swallowing, or who will not move their necks; CT scan may be required for diagnosis; angiography for penetrating injuries to the medial posterior pharynx
- Fine needle aspiration/I&D for peritonsillar abscess

STREP PHARYNGITIS (CONFIRMED)
- Penicillin (250 mg PO TID for children <27 kg and 500 mg PO TID for >27 kg)
- Benzathine penicillin G IM (600,000 U for children <27 kg and 1,200,000 for children >27 kg × 1 dose) or amoxicillin (50 mg/kg daily × 10 days, max dose is 1,000 mg/dL)

FOR PENICILLIN ALLERGIC CHILDREN
- Cephalexin (20 mg/kg/dose BID × 10 days, max dose is 500 mg/dose), cefadroxil (30 mg/kg/dose daily × 10 days, max 1 g), clindamycin (7 mg/kg/dose TID × 10 days, max 300 mg/dose), azithromycin (12 mg/kg/dose, × 5 days, max 500 mg/dose), or clarithromycin (7.5 mg/kg/dose BID × 10 days, max 250 mg/dose)

CONSULT
- ENT for pharyngeal deep neck infection

DICTATION/DOCUMENTATION
- **General:** awake and alert, not toxic appearing
- **VS and SaO$_2$:** fever, tachycardia
- **Skin:** PWD, normal texture and turgor. No pallor or cyanosis. No petechiae, purpura, scarlatiniform rash
- **HEENT:**
  - **Head:** atraumatic, NT, fontanel flat
  - **Eyes:** sclera and conjunctiva clear, PERRLA, EOMI
  - **Ears:** no pre-or postauricular lymphadenopathy or erythema; canals are clear, no erythema, edema, exudates, or foreign body. No cerumen impaction. TMs pearly grey without bulging or retraction. Good light reflex. No fluid level, vesicles, or bullae. No perforation
  - **Nose/Face:** no foreign body, no rhinorrhea, congestion
  - **Mouth/Throat:** Mucous membranes moist and pink, without vesicles, ulcerations, or inflammation. No palatal ulcers or petechiae. No fullness or bulging of posterior soft palate. Uvula midline without edema or erythema. Posterior pharynx clear without lesions, erythema, exudates, or asymmetry. No pain on palpation of jaw or TMJ. No evidence of trauma or foreign body. No drooling
- **Neck:** supple, FROM, nontender, no lymphadenopathy, no meningismus
- **Chest:** CTA
- **Heart:** RRR without murmur
- **Abd:** round, BSA, NT, no HSM
- **Back:** no spinal or CVAT
- **Extremities:** FROM, good strength and tone bilaterally. Neurovascularly intact
- **Neuro:** alert, active, with age-appropriate behavior, GCS 15, no focal neurological findings noted

(cont.)

THROAT PAIN (cont.)

○ TIPS

- Rapid strep test is the preferred diagnostic test to treat strep pharyngitis, if available
- Most cases of uncomplicated pharyngitis are viral

DON'T MISS!

- Deep neck infection, as the airway may become compromised
- Consider epiglottitis or diphtheria in children who are not immunized
- Foreign bodies in the throat or esophagus

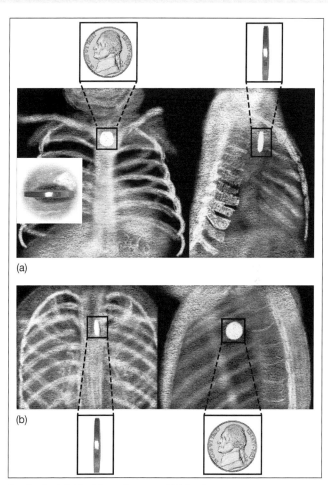

(a)

(b)

Foreign body in the (a) esophagus and (b) trachea

DENTAL/INTRAORAL PAIN

DENTAL TRAUMA

- Concussion: injury to tooth that causes pain; no mobility or displacement
- Subluxation: loosened tooth with blood at gingival sulcus; no displacement
- Extrusion: loosened tooth with partial displacement from socket
- Intrusion: tooth displaced into alveolar bone; associated with fracture of alveolar socket
- Avulsion: tooth completely displaced from socket

FRACTURE CLASSIFICATION

- Ellis I involves only enamel. Teeth stable, NT, no visible color change, rough edges
- Ellis II involves enamel and dentin. Tender to touch and air; visible exposed yellow dentin
- Ellis III involves enamel, dentin, and pulp with visible area of pink, or red, or blood at center of tooth

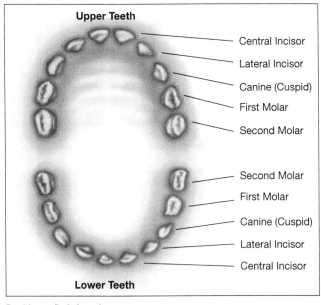

Upper Teeth

Central Incisor
Lateral Incisor
Canine (Cuspid)
First Molar
Second Molar

Second Molar
First Molar
Canine (Cuspid)
Lateral Incisor
Central Incisor

Lower Teeth

Deciduous (baby) teeth

(cont.)

DENTAL/INTRAORAL PAIN (cont.)

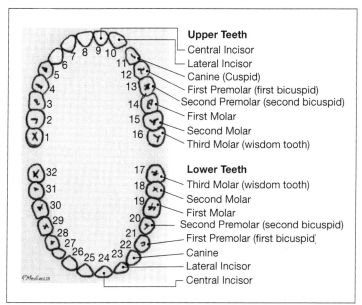

Upper Teeth
Central Incisor
Lateral Incisor
Canine (Cuspid)
First Premolar (first bicuspid)
Second Premolar (second bicuspid)
First Molar
Second Molar
Third Molar (wisdom tooth)

Lower Teeth
Third Molar (wisdom tooth)
Second Molar
First Molar
Second Premolar (second bicuspid)
First Premolar (first bicuspid)
Canine
Lateral Incisor
Central Incisor

Adult teeth chart

HX

- Pain, swelling, temperature sensitivity, fever, difficulty swallowing, breathing, opening mouth
- Time of injury: delayed presentation, extent of tooth avulsion time
- Where did the injury occur: possibility and degree of contamination
- MOI: fall on chin may be associated with crown or crown–root dental fracture
- Pain with exposure to heat or cold: concern for exposed dentin or pulp
- Altered bite, jaw pain
- LOC, associated injuries
- Orthodontia, protective teeth guard, face mask, helmet

(cont.)

DENTAL/INTRAORAL PAIN (cont.)

PE

- **General:** use default
- **VS and SaO$_2$**
- **Skin:** PWD
- **Facial:** swelling, neck swelling/lymphadenopathy
- **Mouth/Throat:** use default
- **Teeth:** normal, broken, or decayed teeth, gingival swelling and erythema, tender to percussion, braces. Primary or permanent teeth involved
  - **Periodontal:** involves tissue surrounding the teeth
  - **Periapical:** infection at root of tooth caused by caries. Often presents with facial swelling, fever, and malaise. Requires root canal or extraction. May extend to periosteum. May see small draining fistula on gingiva of periapical abscess tooth (parulis)
  - **Pericoronal:** tissue over impacted tooth inflamed and infected; tooth not involved
- **Molar infections with spread to mandibular areas**
- **Swelling:**
  - **Sublingual:** swelling of floor of mouth, possible elevation of tongue
  - **Submental:** midline induration under chin
  - **Submandibular:** tenderness and swelling of angle of jaw, trismus
  - **Retropharyngeal space:** sore throat with normal exam, pain, stiff neck, dysphagia, hot potato voice, stridor
  - **Ludwig's angina:** brawny, board-like induration of soft tissues of anterior neck rapidly cause airway compromise
- **Upper teeth infections:** facial swelling at nasolabial fold. May extend to infraorbital area and cause cavernous sinus thrombosis (headache, fever, periorbital swelling, chemosis/bloody chemosis, visual changes)
- **Dry socket (alveolar osteitis):** severe pain, foul odor, grayish debris at socket 4 to 5 days after extraction. Gentle cleansing, sedative dressing, such as oil of cloves, analgesia
- **Gingivitis:** inflammation of gum tissue, ANUG: swollen, red gums with ulcers, foul odor, easy bleeding, devitalized tissue
- **Sialolithiasis (duct stone):** Wharton's duct—submandibular, Stensen's duct—parotid
- **Sialadenitis** ductal inflammation or infection

(cont.)

DENTAL/INTRAORAL PAIN (cont.)

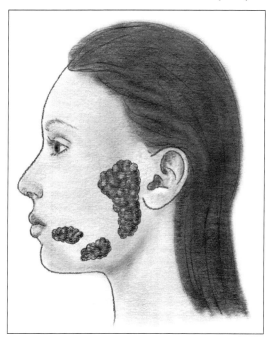

The locations of the salivary duct glands

MDM/DDx

Toddlers are at risk for frequent falls as they learn to walk and become more mobile. Older children may be injured in sports, falls, MVCs, or altercations. **Facial trauma** that causes dental injuries can lead to functional or cosmetic problems and sometimes psychological trauma. Decisions to treat injured primary teeth are based on the age and viability of the tooth; extraction may be performed and a temporary tooth inserted. **Dental trauma** resulting in complete **tooth avulsion** is a dental emergency and can lead to tooth loss caused by root resorption. **Dental infections** can be painful and can spread to adjacent facial or periorbital soft tissues or sinuses. Although not common in children, severe infections can cause potential airway compromise caused by **retropharyngeal space infection** or **Ludwig's angina. Dry socket** (alveolar osteitis) is a painful condition that can occur 4 to 5 days after dental extraction. Red, inflamed, swollen gum tissue indicates **gingivitis** that can be treated by appropriate brushing and flossing. Consider aggressive periodontitis in adolescents with marked inflammation and heavy plaque. Excess intraoral bacteria can lead to **ANUG**, which causes foul breath, easy bleeding, and necrotic tissue. This very painful disease may be found in debilitated or immunosuppressed children or those with malnutrition or poor oral hygiene. Ductal stones **(sialolithiasis)** are not common in children but may present with pain while eating

(cont.)

DENTAL/INTRAORAL PAIN (cont.)

MANAGEMENT

- **Infection:** dental and intraoral infections often caused by polymicrobial organisms; treat with 7 to 10 days course of Abx
  - PVK 500 mg PO QID; amoxicillin/clavulanate 875 PO BID; clindamycin 300 to 450 mg. PVK 25 to 50 mg/kg/d in equally divided doses TID; amoxicillin/clavulanate 25 to 45 mg/kg in two divided doses; clindamycin 8 to 25 mg/kg/d in three divided doses PO or IV; ampicillin/sulbactam 100 to 400 mg/kg/d up q6h up to a maximum of 8 g/d PO TID; or clindamycin 600 to 900 mg IV TID or ampicillin/sulbactam 3 g IV q6h
- **Concussion** and **subluxation:** analgesia, local rinsing, advise soft foods, observe. Refer subluxation for possible flexible splint for comfort. **Extrusion:** gently manually straighten and reinsert into socket; refer for splinting. **Intrusion:** prophylactic Abx and refer for definitive management. **Avulsion:** handle by crown, avoid touching root, rinse. Replant immediately if possible and have pt bite on gauze to stabilize; or place in saliva, milk, Hank's solution, saline (no water)
- **Dry socket (alveolar osteitis):** gentle cleansing, sedative dressing such as oil of cloves, analgesia
- **Ductal stones:** possible Ultz or CT for identification, increase salivation with sour candies, Abx if infected

⊙ TIPS

- Exposed pulp is normal when hot/cold stimuli is sensed; lack of response to stimulus increases risk of later pulp necrosis
- Be wary of dental infections in pts with diabetes, chemotherapy with neutropenia
- Watch for airway compromise, sepsis, Ludwig's angina

NECK/CERVICAL PAIN/INJURY

HX

- Onset, location, duration, characteristics
- F/C, N/V
- Aggravating/relieving factors
- Treatments used, OTC pain meds
- Time and circumstances of pain/injury
- MOI: flexion, extension, rotation, lateral flexion, axial loading
- Blunt or penetrating trauma (type and direction of weapon)
- Sports, assault, diving, seizure
- MVC/motorcycle (speed, seat belt, location in vehicle, airbag deployment, extent of car damage, ejection, extrication)
- Serious MVC, unrestrained, auto versus pedestrian, fatality at scene
- Fall >3 ft or >5 steps or >3 × child's ht
- Choking or hanging. Suicide/homicide
- Concern for basilar skull FX, skull penetration
- Large scalp hematoma
- SCIWORA: neuro deficit on scene with transient resolution and then paralysis
- LOC or ALOC: gradual or sudden, brief lucid interval
- Painful or difficulty speaking, hoarse, drooling
- Headache, visual changes, face/neck pain, seizure, N/V
- Blood/CSF leak from nose/ears
- Spinal or extremity pain, numbness, tingling, weakness
- Drugs, ETOH
- Distracting injury (e.g., extremity injury)

(cont.)

NECK/CERVICAL PAIN/INJURY (cont.)

PE
- **General:** position of pt (e.g., spinal precautions), level of distress; ALOC, irritable, lethargic
- **VS and SaO$_2$:** bradycardia and hypotension indicate neurogenic shock; hypothermia caused by poikilothermia (inability to regulate core temperature)
- **Skin:** warm, dry, flushed skin (neurogenic shock), cap refill
- **HEENT:**
    - **Head:** scalp contusion, tenderness, open wounds, FB, bony step-off or deformity
    - **Eyes:** PERRLA, EOMI, subconjunctival hemorrhage, petechiae, periorbital ecchymosis
    - **Ears:** Battle's sign, hemotympanum, CSF leak
    - **Nose/Face:** septal hematoma, epistaxis, CSF rhinorrhea, facial petechiae, TTP, symmetry, trauma
    - **Mouth/Throat:** drooling, hoarseness, stridor, intraoral bleeding; teeth and mandible
- **Neck:** surface trauma, open wounds, soft tissue or muscle tenderness, trachea midline, tenderness over larynx; subcutaneous emphysema or crepitus. Bony TTP, step-off or deformity to firm palpation at posterior midline. FROM without limitation or pain, flexion, extension, lateral bending, rotation, and axial load
- **Chest:** surface trauma, symmetry, tenderness, hypoventilation, lung sounds, tachypnea or bradypnea, hemoptysis
- **Heart:** RRR, normal tones, no murmurs, rubs, or gallops
- **Abd:** surface trauma, BSA, tenderness, guarding, rigidity, bladder distension
- **Back:** surface trauma, spinal or CVAT
- **GU:** femoral pulses; priapism (involuntary erection occurs with high cervical cord injury), urinary retention
- **Rectal:** saddle anesthesia, anal wink, sphincter tone, fecal incontinence
- **Extremities:** FROM, NT, distal CMS intact; assess proximal and distal muscle strength and sensation and compare to other side
- **Neuro:** A&O ×3, GCS 15, CN II–XII, no focal neuro deficits, grip strength, reflex strength or flaccid, bulbocavernosus reflex (monitor rectal sphincter tone in response to gentle tug on urinary catheter or squeeze glans penis), Babinski reflex (abnormal extension of toes)

MDM/DDx

Many children complain of neck pain due to benign or self-limiting problems such as **torticollis** (wry neck) caused by sleeping wrong or lateral twisting of the neck or mild **muscle strain** or **spasm**. These problems do not involve upper extremity paresthesia. More serious injuries are **ligamentous injury, fracture,** or **subluxation**. It is possible to have a **spinal cord injury without radiographic abnormality. Spinal cord injury** must be considered in every pt presenting with C/O of neck pain. Emergent findings are flaccid paralysis, loss of bowel and bladder reflexes and tone, and hemodynamic instability. Overlooked spine injuries can have devastating effects and suspicion for serious injury based on mechanism of injury is essential. Medication-induced **dystonic reactions** are more common in children who are ill or dehydrated. **Cervical lymphadenopathy** can occur as an isolated node or regionally. Inflamed and enlarged lymph nodes can be the result of a focal infection of the ear, teeth, or throat. Also consider **cat scratch fever (subacute regional lymphadenitis)** if there is a HX of cat scratch/bite in the previous few weeks. Neck pain with a normal posterior pharynx exam should prompt investigation for more serious etiologies that can cause airway problems such as **severe pharyngitis/tonsillitis, peritonsillar abscess,** or **retropharyngeal abscess**

(cont.)

NECK/CERVICAL PAIN/INJURY (cont.)

MANAGEMENT

▨ ABCs, spinal immobilization, ice, nonsteroidal anti-inflammatory drugs (NSAIDs), opioids (steroids controversial)
▨ **C-spine criteria:** evidence-based criteria used to "clear" pt with potential cervical spine injury without radiographs
   ▨ No posterior midline cervical spine tenderness
   ▨ No evidence of intoxication is present
   ▨ Normal level of alertness
   ▨ No focal neurologic deficit is present
   ▨ No painful distracting injury
   ▨ FROM on flexion, extension, and lateral bending
▨ **Cross-table lateral view is not sufficient to clear a C-spine**
   ▨ C-spine x-ray (three or five view)
▨ CT of neck based on MOI
▨ Must be able to visualize all C1–C7 to T1 vertebrae; MRI for ligamentous injury

DICTATION/DOCUMENTATION

▨ **General:** use default and state position of pt (e.g., full spinal precautions), level of distress/pain. Awake and alert in no distress; no odor of ETOH
▨ **VS and SaO$_2$**
▨ **Skin:** PWD, no surface trauma
▨ **HEENT:**
   ▨ **Head:** traumatic, no palpable soft tissue or bony deformities. Fontanel flat (if still open)
   ▨ **Eyes:** PERRLA, EOMI, no subconjunctival hemorrhage, petechiae, periorbital ecchymosis
   ▨ **Ears:** TMs clear, no hemotympanum or Battle's sign
   ▨ **Nose/Face:** atraumatic, no asymmetry, no epistaxis or septal hematoma. Facial bones symmetric, NT to palpation, and stable with attempts at manipulation
   ▨ **Mouth/Throat:** voice clear, no pain with speaking; no drooling or stridor; no intra-oral trauma, teeth and mandible are intact
▨ **Neck:** no surface trauma, open wounds, soft tissue or muscle tenderness or spasm; trachea midline, no tenderness over larynx. No subQ emphysema or crepitus. No bony tenderness, step-off, or deformity to firm palpation at posterior midline. FROM without limitation or pain; normal flexion, extension, lateral bending, rotation, and axial load
▨ **Chest:** no surface trauma or asymmetry. NT without crepitus or deformity. Normal tidal volume. CTA bilaterally. SaO$_2$ >94% WNL
▨ **Heart:** RRR. Tones are normal. All peripheral pulses are intact and equal
▨ **Abd:** nondistended without abrasions or ecchymosis. BSA, soft, NT, guarding, or rebound. No masses. Good femoral pulses
▨ **Back:** NT without step-off or deformity to firm palpation of the thoracic and lumbar spine. No contusions, ecchymosis, or abrasions are noted
▨ **GU:** Normal external genitalia with no blood at the meatus (if applicable). No priapism
▨ **Pelvis:** NT to palpation and stable to compression
▨ **Rectal:** normal tone. No rectal wall tenderness or mass. Stool is brown and heme negative (if applicable)
▨ **Extremities:** no surface trauma. FROM. Distal motor, neurovascular supply is intact
▨ **Neuro:** A&O ×3, GCS 15, CN II–XII grossly intact. C/M/S intact. No focal neuro deficits

(cont.)

NECK/CERVICAL PAIN/INJURY (cont.)

◯ TIP

- C2 vertebra most commonly injured followed by C6 and C7 injury

DON'T MISS!

- Flaccid, no reflexes, loss of anal sphincter tone, incontinence, priapism
- Hypotension; bradycardia; flushed, dry, and warm skin
- Ileus, urinary retention, poikilothermia
- SCIWORA
- **Neuro level:**
- **C6** = palmar surface of thumb, index, 1/2 of the third finger
- **C7** = palmar surface of third finger
- **C8** = palmar surface of fourth and fifth fingers

COUGH/SOB

HX

- Onset sudden or gradual, duration of cough or SOB
- Cough wet versus dry, barking, whooping/spasms, choking, nocturnal, associated with feeding, hemoptysis, posttussive emesis
- Wheezing, grunting, including WOB, retractions
- Sputum production—color, amount, consistency
- FB ingestion suspected or known
- F/C, N/V
- "Spitting up," "wet burps," dry heaves, fussiness during and after feeding
- Chest pain, abd pain, dizziness
- Fatigue, malaise
- Dyspnea, periods of apnea or bradypnea, orthopnea, cyanosis, PND
- Postnasal drip/sinus congestion
- Change in voice (muffled or hoarse)
- Smoke exposure, environmental irritants, travel, sick contacts
- Night sweats, weight loss
- HIV/TB risk factors
- IVDA or illicit drug use (e.g., cocaine)
- Trauma
- HX: prematurity, cardiopulmonary disease (e.g., BPD, CF, congenital heart disease), congenital anomalies, previous episodes, hospitalizations/intubation, steroids, home O_2, ALTE, GERD
- FH: asthma, cancer, connective tissue disease
- Immunizations, medications
- Hospitalizations for respiratory-related illnesses, last steroid use, intubations

PE

- **General:** F/C, restlessness, anxiety, somnolence, lethargy
- **VS and SaO$_2$:** tachypnea, tachycardia, pulsus paradoxus
- **Skin:** rash, ashen, cyanosis, pallor
- **HEENT:**
  - **Head:** normocephalic, atraumatic, bobbing
  - **Eyes:** discharge, edema, erythema, allergic shiners
  - **Ears:** TMs and canals clear
  - **Nose:** rhinorrhea, flare, snoring, boggy, hyperemic, sinuses TTP/erythema
  - **Mouth/Throat:** MMM, halitosis, erythema, exudate, stridor, drooling
- **Neck:** supple, FROM, lymphadenopathy, meningismus, JVD
- **Chest:** WOB, effort, retractions, accessory muscle use, grunting, Kussmaul, paradoxical abd breathing. CTA, wheezes, crackles, rhonchi, pleural friction rub, orthopnea, sniffing, or tripod position, able to speak easily in full sentences
- **Heart:** RRR, no murmurs, rubs, or gallops
- **Abd:** soft, BSA, NT
- **Extremities:** FROM, good strength and tone, neurovascularly intact or STS, edema, status of upper extremity circulation
- **Neuro:** alert, active, with age appropriate behavior, GCS 15, no focal neurologic deficit

(cont.)

COUGH/SOB (cont.)

MDM/DDx

The most common cause of acute cough in children is **viral upper respiratory infection** with or without **bronchospasm**. Cough in infants 2 months of age and younger is more likely to be more serious than in the older age groups. In infants and young children, tachypnea, retractions, and decreased effort are key indicators of respiratory distress that can lead to respiratory failure and/or arrest. **Neonatal apnea** and bradypnea are usually the result of central immaturity or respiratory fatigue. An **ALTE** is an episode in which there is some combination of apnea (central or obstructive), color change (e.g., cyanosis, erythematous), change in muscle tone, and choking/gagging episode. Other causes of **apnea** include abusive head trauma, metabolic acidosis, and poisoning. **Tracheomalacia** is characterized by a harsh noise/stridor on expiration early in the neonatal period. **Bronchiolitis** is manifested by fever, nasal congestion, wheezing, cough and crackles, nasal flaring, retractions, and tachypnea. The cough associated with **croup** is a hoarse, barky cough, worse at night, stridor, and possible respiratory distress. Typical findings in **pneumonia** include fever, cough, wheezing, focal crackles, decreased breath sounds, and retractions. Fever is usually absent in **atypical pneumonia**. **Chlamydia pneumonia** usually manifests itself within the first 2 weeks of life, and may be associated with conjunctivitis, staccato cough, and absence of fever. The cough of **pertussis** may be associated with the characteristic whoop. However, infants are usually not capable of generating enough force and may present with cyanosis and apnea. **Reactive airway disease** with bronchospasm may present with cough with or without wheezing, tachypnea, retractions, and respiratory distress. Older children with bronchospasm and wheezing may have **asthma** that is exacerbated by viral infections, exercise, or irritants. Upper **airway obstruction** (e.g., foreign body aspiration) is manifested by choking, gagging, changes in voice, stridor. Infants and toddlers have immature control of the airway and are at risk for lower airway aspiration; suspect if history of choking, persistent cough, new onset of wheezing. Passage of gastric contents into the esophagus can lead to simple gastroesophageal reflux (**GERD**) or cause actual GERD. It is common in infants with immature lower esophageal sphincters and usually resolves by age 1 year. Consider GERD in children with more serious symptoms such as discomfort, persistent cough, regurgitation, heartburn, or poor weight gain

(cont.)

COUGH/SOB (cont.)

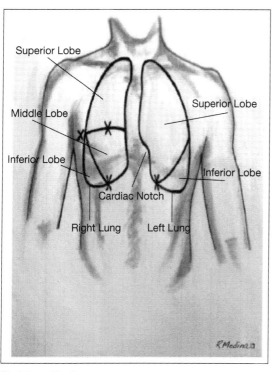

The lobes of the lungs
Source: Adapted from Fine, M. J., Auble, T. E., Yealy, D. M., Hanusa,
B. H., Weissfeld, L. A., Singer, D. E., . . . Kapoor, W. N. (1997). A prediction
rule to identify low-risk patients with community acquired pneumonia.
New England Journal of Medicine, 336, 243–250. doi:10.1056/NEJM
199701233360402

(cont.)

COUGH/SOB (cont.)

MANAGEMENT

- **Labs:** CBC with differential, BMP, ESR, CRP, and blood culture if infection is suspected and child is ill appearing. ABG or VBG. Nasal swab, pertussis culture, or PCR
- **Imaging:** soft tissue lateral neck x-ray may identify tracheitis, epiglottis, croup, or a radiopaque foreign body. AP and lateral CXR can localize and identify pulmonary consolidation, atelectasis, pleural and/or pericardial fluid, and air leak but may have a false negative result; lateral decubitus CXR may be useful in identifying a foreign body aspiration. Lung ultz may have more sensitivity and specificity to identify pediatric pneumonia and may be ordered based on local practice and availability
- **Viral URI:** supportive care, fever control, fluids
- **Bronchiolitis:** provide supplemental oxygen if hypoxic SaO$_2$ <90%, trial of inhaled bronchodilator for moderate to severe respiratory distress (e.g., nasal flaring; retractions; grunting; respiratory rate >70 breaths per minute; dyspnea; or cyanosis), fluids (IV or PO if tolerated)
- **Croup:** Decadron (0.6 mg/kg, maximum of 10 mg) by the least invasive route possible: PO, IM, or IV. With moderate stridor at rest and moderate retractions, or more severe symptoms administer racemic epinephrine as 0.05 mL/kg per dose (maximum of 0.5 mL) of a 2.25% solution diluted to 3 mL total volume with normal saline via nebulizer over 15 minutes. Racemic epinephrine can be repeated every 15 to 20 minutes. Children who have received racemic epinephrine should be observed for at least 3 hours and then may be discharged if there is no stridor at rest
- **Pneumonia:** in afebrile infants <4 months of age with CAP, the most likely bacterial pathogen is *C. trachomatis* and should be treated with erythromycin (50 mg/kg/d in four divided doses for 14 days). High-dose amoxicillin (80–90 mg/kg per day divided into two or three doses; maximum dose 4 g/d) should be used in older children with CAP. A second- or third-generation cephalosporin is an alternate choice
- **Reactive airway disease with bronchospasm/asthma:** inhaled bronchodilator (albuterol 2.5–5.0 mg/dose Q10–20 min PRN or 15 to 20 mg/dose over 1 hour continuous nebulizer) with Atrovent 500 mcg/dose. Methylprednisolone or prednisone 1 to 2 mg/kg/dose. Magnesium IV (50 mg/kg/dose 2 g maximum dose). Terbutaline (0.01 mg/kg SC). Supplemental oxygen to maintain SaO$_2$ > 93%. Heliox (80/20) for continued respiratory distress
- **Pertussis:** azithromycin (10 mg/kg/d for 5 days), erythromycin (10 mg/kg/d four times a day for 14 days), trimethoprim/sulfamethoxazole (8 to 12 mg TMP/kg/d in divided doses every 12 hours; maximum single dose: 160 mg TMP)
- **GERD:** in infants is usually benign and managed with parental education regarding small, frequent feedings, positioning child upright after feeding for 20 min, and elevated HOB in crib. GERD can be diagnosed with esophageal pH and a trial of acid-suppressive medication. Imaging may include barium swallow/upper GI series or endoscopy. Meds that may improve GERD SXS include Mylicon or Gaviscon, Mylanta/Maalox, H2 blockers (ranitidine, famotidine, cimetidine), or PPIs (omeprazole, lansoprazole, rabeprazole), but use with caution

(cont.)

COUGH/SOB (cont.)

DICTATION/DOCUMENTATION

- **General:** awake and alert, in no obvious resp distress
- **VS and SaO$_2$**
- **Skin:** PWD, no cyanosis or pallor
- **HEENT:**
  - **Head:** normocephalic
  - **Eyes:** PERRLA, sclera and conjunctiva clear
  - **Ears:** canals and TMs normal
  - **Nose:** no rhinorrhea or nasal flare
  - **Mouth/Throat:** MMM, posterior pharynx clear
- **Neck:** supple, FROM, no JVD, trachea midline
- **Chest:** no orthopnea or dyspnea. Able to speak in complete sentences, no retractions or accessory muscle use, no tripod position. Infants: no grunting, stridor, or head bobbing. CTA, no wheezes, rhonchi, crackles
- **Heart:** RRR
- **Abd:** soft, BSA, nondistended. NT. No masses or HSM
- **Back:** no spinal or CVAT
- **Extremities:** FROM, good strength and tone bilaterally. Neurovascularly intact. No swelling/edema, NT
- **Neuro:** alert, active, with age-appropriate behavior, GCS 15, no focal neurologic deficit

CXR INTERPRETATION NOTE

Note whether one- or two-view chest film done; no bony abnormality (i.e., no DJD, lytic lesions, rib FX); heart is normal size, no cardiomegaly; lungs reveal no pneumothorax, hyperinflation, infiltrate, effusion, mass, cavitation (TB), or FB aspiration; mediastinum not widened, no pneumomediastinum, and no hilar adenopathy or tracheal deviation

⊘ TIPS

- Bronchiolitis can cause apnea in up to 20% of infants
- Wheezing in infants may indicate congenital heart disease
- Foreign body aspiration in infants or toddlers

DON'T MISS!

- Child maltreatment as a cause of apnea

CHEST PAIN

HX

- P = Provoking/precipitating factors; alleviating factors
- Q = Quality—sharp, heavy, achy, tight, tearing
- R = Radiation/region—migration or movement of pain, localized or diffuse
- S = Severity—pain scale 1 to 10, face scale
- T = Timing of onset, sudden versus gradual, acute versus chronic, duration, time of day, exercise induced
- Back/flank pain, abd/epigastric pain
- Painful swallowing, heartburn, hematemesis, melena
- SOB, exertional dyspnea, F/C, N/V, indigestion
- Diaphoresis, dizziness, syncope, cough, hemoptysis
- Fatigue, malaise, fever, vomiting
- Recent viral illness or surgical procedures
- Recurrent somatic complaints
- FH: sudden cardiac death of first-degree relative, connective tissue disease (e.g., Marfan syndrome)
- SH: smoke exposure, ETOH, illicit drug use, recent stressful life events, recent increase in physical activity
- HX: congenital heart disease, sickle cell disease, asthma, Kawasaki disease, obesity, previous EKG
- Risk factors for maltreatment/interpersonal/family violence (see "Maltreatment")
- Risk factors for PE (rare in children): sickle cell disease, congenital heart disease, central venous lines, neoplasm, conditions with reduced protein synthesis, trauma, DVT

PE

- **General:** position of pt, level of distress
- **VS and SaO$_2$:** fever, tachycardia, irregularity, BP both arms
- **Skin:** pale, cool, diaphoretic, cyanosis
- **HEENT:**
    - **Head:** normocephalic
    - **Eyes:** pupils PERRLA and EOMI
    - **Ears:** TMs and canals clear
    - **Nose:** patent
    - **Mouth/Throat:** MMM
- **Neck:** FROM, trachea midline, bruits, JVD, subcutaneous emphysema
- **Chest:** NT, WOB, retractions, accessory muscle use, TTP, CTA, wheezes, crackles, rhonchi, pleural friction rub (bruising, rib, scapular, or sternal FXs—require force)
- **Heart:** RRR, no murmur, gallop, rub, muffled, clear tones
- **Abd:** SNT, epigastric mass, pulsation; stool OB
- **Extremities:** STS, edema, status of upper extremity circulation, femoral pulses (e.g., cardiac problems in infants), erythema, skin discoloration, warmth, tenderness. FROM, good strength and tone bilaterally. Neurovascularly intact
- **Neuro:** alert, active, with age-appropriate behavior, GCS 15, no focal neurological findings

(cont.)

CHEST PAIN (cont.)

MDM/DDx

Most causes of chest pain in children are benign. **Musculoskeletal pain** is the most common etiology and is usually atraumatic. **Costochondritis** is typically unilateral tenderness of the costal cartilage, most commonly on the left side. **Myalgias** of the chest wall may also occur, commonly referred to as **chest wall syndrome.** Body position movement and deep breathing may exacerbate musculoskeletal pain. **Respiratory disorders**, including pneumonia, bronchitis, and reactive airway disease, are also common causes of chest pain. **Exercise-induced bronchoconstriction** can lead to chest pain, even in pts without audible wheezing. **Gastrointestinal disorders** that can cause chest pain include disorders of the esophagus (most common), stomach, bowel, biliary tract, and pancreas. Inflammatory conditions of the heart (endocarditis, myocarditis, or pericarditis) require a high index of suspicion as nonspecific prodromal symptoms may be overlooked. The cardiac exam varies with the underlying pathology and specific site of inflammation/infection. **Endocarditis** is characterized by prolonged flu-like symptoms, fever, weight loss, possible new regurgitant murmur, and extra-cardiac symptoms (arthritis, neurologic deficits, hematuria, Osler's nodes, Roth's spots, splenomegaly). **Myocarditis** is characterized by pleuritic or precordial stabbing chest pain, flu-like symptoms, and a new murmur. The pain of **pericarditis** is sometimes reproduced with direct pressure to the sternal region and improves with sitting up and leaning forward. Serious underlying organic medical conditions, including cardiac disease, are rare but potentially dangerous. **Cardiac disease** is more likely if the pain occurs during exertion and is recurrent. Associated symptoms include palpitations and syncope. **Acute chest syndrome** is a potentially fatal cause of chest pain with **sickle cell disease** (see "Sickle Cell Disease") and occurs in almost 50% of this pt population. ACS is associated with a new pulmonary infiltrate involving at least one complete lung segment, fever, tachypnea, wheezing, or cough. **Psychogenic causes** are also a common etiology of chest pain in children, although more common in adolescents. Suspect **maltreatment** with **chest bruising, abrasions, contusions, rib FXs, pneumothorax,** injuries in different stages of healing, and/or injuries that are inconsistent with the MOI. Less common causes of chest pain include **pleuritis, pleural effusion, pneumothorax, pulmonary embolism, and pneumomediastinum** (resulting from trauma, reactive airway disease, cystic fibrosis, or Marfan syndrome)

MANAGEMENT

- EKG if cardiac disease is suspected, abnormal pulse rate, palpitations, or syncope
- CXR if cardiac or pulmonary disease is suspected. Lung ultz may have more sensitivity and specificity to identify pediatric thoracic abnormalities and may be ordered based on local practice and availability
- CBC, ESR, CRP, BMP, urinary pregnancy test, possible urine drug screen
- Analgesics (NSAIDs) and rest for musculoskeletal pain
- Bronchodilators and steroids for bronchospasm
- Pediatric cardiology consult if concern for underlying heart disease

(cont.)

CHEST PAIN (cont.)

DICTATION/DOCUMENTATION

- **General:** awake and alert, in no obvious distress
- **VS and SaO$_2$:** BP both arms
- **Skin:** PWD, no diaphoresis, cyanosis, or pallor
- **HEENT:**
  - **Head:** normocephalic
  - **Eyes:** PERRLA, sclera and conjunctiva clear
  - **Ears:** canals and TMs normal
  - **Nose:** patent
  - **Mouth/Throat:** MMM, posterior pharynx clear
- **Neck:** supple, FROM, no JVD, trachea midline, no bruits
- **Chest:** no orthopnea or dyspnea noted; no retractions or accessory muscle use. NT, no crepitus. CTA bilaterally, no wheezes, rhonchi, crackles
- **Heart:** RRR, no murmur, gallop, rub
- **Abd:** soft, BSA, NT, no epigastric tenderness, mass, pulsation; femoral pulses
- **Back:** no CVAT
- **Extremities:** FROM, good strength and tone bilaterally. No swelling, edema, tenderness. Neurovascularly intact
- **Neuro:** alert, active, with age-appropriate behavior, GCS 15, no LOC and no focal neurological deficits

◗ TIPS

- Suspect maltreatment with
  - Chest bruising, abrasions, contusions, rib FXs, pneumothorax injuries in different stages of healing
  - Injuries inconsistent with the MOI

DON'T MISS!

Serious causes of chest pain in children:
- Ischemia (e.g., Kawasaki's)
- Acute chest syndrome
- Pulmonary (emboli, pneumothorax)
- Arrhythmias
- Infections (pericarditis, myocarditis, endocarditis)

CONGENITAL HEART DISEASE

HX

- Depends on etiology
- Most common presentation is respiratory distress and cyanotic episodes
- Signs of CHF include pallor, fatigue, tachypnea, increased respiratory effort at rest or during feeding, irritability, dehydration, poor appetite, diaphoresis during feeding, S3 heart sound, hepatomegaly, failure to thrive, recurrent lung infections

PE

- **General:** alert, active, lethargic
- **VS and SaO$_2$:** tachycardia, tachypnea. BP measured in arm and leg, SaO$_2$ measured in right hand and either foot
- **Skin:** cyanotic, pallor, pink, warm, dry, cool
- **HEENT:** dysmorphic features, head bobbing, nasal flaring
- **Chest:** persistent tachypnea, increased respiratory effort at rest, grunting, retractions, chest congestion
- **Heart:** murmurs with or without trills, S3
- **Abd:** hepatomegaly
- **Extremities:** cool or mottled; absent or decreased distal pulses
- **Neuro:** alert, active, with age-appropriate behavior, GCS 15, no focal neurological findings

MDM/DDx

Clinical presentation can vary from asymptomatic, cyanotic, **congestive heart failure**, to **cardiogenic shock**. Two typical age groups: **ductal-dependent lesions** present in first month of life; left to right shunt lesions present in the 2- to 6-month age group. Undiagnosed pts can present in extremis at any age. **Central cyanosis** indicates R to L shunt; pallor indicates outflow obstruction, systemic hypoperfusion, and shock. Cyanosis may not be detectable until the SaO$_2$ is <80% in a newborn. Cool skin and delayed capillary refill indicate shock. Blood pressure 10 mmHg or higher in the arms than the legs is clinically significant. Difference in SaO$_2$ between right hand and lower extremity >3% to 5% is clinically significant. **Sepsis** must be considered in neonates. Other diagnostic considerations include **hypoglycemia**, persistent **pulmonary hypertension, ALTE, pneumonia, inborn errors of metabolism,** dilated **cardiomyopathy, myocarditis, arrhythmias,** and **structural heart disease**

MANAGEMENT

- **Immediate stabilization, ABCs,** continuous pulse oximetry; administer O$_2$ judiciously; IV access with small, frequent boluses of 10 mL/kg to treat hypotension; stat glucose level
- **Lab:** CBC (polycythemia or anemia may be present); serum electrolytes (hyponatremia, hypochloremia); calcium (hypocalcemia); glucose (hypoglycemia); cardiac enzymes (CPK-MB, troponin); blood culture; ABG (hypoxemia, metabolic acidosis)
- **Imaging:** CXR is essential (heart can be small, normal, or large); lung ultz may have more sensitivity and specificity to identify pediatric thoracic abnormalities and may be ordered based on local practice and availability
- **Diagnostic procedures:** 12-lead or 15-lead EKG, echocardiogram, hyperoxia test (differentiates cardiac vs. pulmonary disease)
- **Other:** empiric antibiotics if sepsis is suspected, PGE1 infusion (ductal-dependent CHD); furosemide, dopamine, dobutamine

(cont.)

CONGENITAL HEART DISEASE (cont.)

DICTATION/DOCUMENTATION

- **General:** well-developed infant; warm, dry, and pink
- **VS and SaO$_2$**
- **HEENT:**
  - **Head:** normocephalic, anterior, and posterior fontanels flat
  - **Eyes:** sclera white, conjunctiva pink, PERRL, red reflex present bilaterally
  - **Ears:** normal position, TMs clear with good light reflex
  - **Nose:** absent nasal flaring, mucosa pink without lesions or discharge
  - **Mouth/Throat:** mucosa and lips pink and moist, uvula midline, hard and soft palate intact, strong cry
- **Chest:** moves symmetrically without increased work of breathing, no grunting or retractions, lungs CTA bilaterally
- **Heart:** RRR + S1, S2, S3, S4 without murmurs, heaves, or trills
- **Abd:** soft, NT, without masses, no hepatosplenomegaly
- **Extremities:** symmetrical movement without deformity, symmetrical muscle tone and strength, no cyanosis or clubbing; upper and lower distal pulses palpable and symmetrical
- **Neuro:** alert, active, with age-appropriate behavior, GCS 15, no focal neurological findings

⊙ TIPS

- Admit for increased O$_2$ requirement over baseline, respiratory distress, worsening CHF
- High concentrations of O$_2$ may worsen a pt with cyanotic CHD. Specialized pediatric critical transport team may be required

DON'T MISS!

- Emergency pediatric cardiology consult

ABDOMINAL PAIN

HX

- Onset: sudden or gradual, pain within 14 days of onset of menstrual cycle, consider PID: localized or diffuse
- Duration: hours to days is more urgent, exacerbation of chronic problem
- Characteristics: intermittent, sharp, dull, achy pain; intermittent or constant, radiation of pain, or pain localized away from midline
- Aggravating/relieving factors/OTC treatments (e.g., home remedies)
- F/C, N/V: number of episodes; bilious; bloody, undigested food; projectile, posttussive vomiting
- Tolerating oral fluids, appetite, wet diapers
- Stools, bowel changes/habits, bloating, passing gas, diarrhea frequency, color, blood, pus, currant-jelly stool
- Flank pain, urinary urgency, frequency, burning pain, hematuria, incontinence
- Referred pain to groin/scrotum, right or left scapula
- Cough, chest pain, or pressure
- PMH: DM, CA, GB, pancreatitis, obesity, connective tissue disease (e.g., Marfan's syndrome)
- PSH: abd surgeries
- FH: PUD or IBD
- Sexual HX, LNMP, vaginal bleeding/discharge
- HX of same pain with new progression, STI: consider PID
- Testicular, groin, back pain
- Recent trauma (maltreatment vs. accidental); MOI (blunt vs. penetrating) assault, fall, MVC, auto/ped, stabbing, GSW, missile injury
- ETOH, tobacco, drugs
- Time of last food and fluid intake
- Recent travel
- Growth disturbance

(cont.)

ABDOMINAL PAIN (cont.)

PE

- ▓ **General:** alert, interactive, able to focus, irritable, lethargic, writhing, still
- ▓ **VS and SaO$_2$:** fever, tachycardia, hypotension
- ▓ **Skin:** PWD or pale, cool, moist; jaundice, dehydration
- ▓ **HEENT:**
  - ▓ **Head:** normocephalic
  - ▓ **Eyes:** sclera icteric; sunken, pupils PERRLA and EOMI
  - ▓ **Ears:** TMs and canals clear
  - ▓ **Nose:** patent
  - ▓ **Mouth/Throat:** MMM
- ▓ **Neck:** supple, no lymphadenopathy, no meningismus, no JVD
- ▓ **Chest:** CTA bilaterally; no crackles, rhonchi, or wheezing
- ▓ **Heart:** RRR, no murmur, gallop, rub
- ▓ **Abd:** soft/flat/distended; BSA, guarding, rebound (able to jump up and down), response to heel tap, rigid, tender, pulsatile masses, scars, surface trauma, hernia, Psoas, and obturator signs
- ▓ **GU:** normal external genitalia, urinary meatus, femoral pulses, no hernia, normal testicles, cremasteric reflex
- ▓ **Rectal:** blood, pain, or mass (fecal impaction, tumor, prostate, pelvic abscess)
- ▓ **Vaginal discharge:** CMT, os closed, no adnexal fullness or TTP
- ▓ **Back:** CVAT, ecchymosis
- ▓ **Extremities:** FROM
- ▓ Include vaginal, testicular, rectal, neuro exam as indicated

MDM/DDx

In spite of many specific etiologies for abd pain, most children are discharged home with a **nonspecific diagnosis.** Pediatric abd pain may be the result of benign and self-limiting causes such as **AGE or mesenteric lymphadenitis.** Priority is on the early identification of pts with potentially life-threatening or surgical causes of abd pain. Normal temperature, hemodynamic stability, and lack of serious comorbidities are reassuring findings. Diagnosis of serious surgical problems, such as **appendicitis, intussusception, volvulus, strangulated hernia,** or **testicular torsion,** is vital. **Intractable pain, uncontrolled vomiting, diarrhea, unstable VS,** or **AMS** in any pt are indications for hospital admission. In children with bilious vomiting and sudden abd pain, consider **malrotation** with midgut volvulus; nonbilious vomiting, consider **hypertrophic pyloric stenosis** (2–12 weeks, up to 20 weeks). Abd pain in "waves," then lethargy, and afebrile, consider **intussusception** (3 months to 6 years; peak incidence 6–12 months). **Diffuse pain:** AGE, DKA, BO, IBD, ischemia, SCD, perforated viscus. Some children with **pneumonia** present with abd pain as chief complaint. **Renal calculi** are less common in children and there is usually an underlying condition. Metabolic problems like **DKA** can present with vague, diffuse abd pain, and vomiting. Underlying inflammatory etiologies, such as **SLE or HSP,** are often associated with complaints of abd pain. **RUQ:** GB, FHCS, hepatitis, PNA, pyelonephritis, renal calculi (late pregnancy with appendicitis—pt may not have RUQ nor classic RLQ pain). **LUQ:** spleen, gastritis, PUD, PNA, pyelonephritis, renal calculi. **RLQ:** appy, renal calc, inguinal hernia, GYN (menses, PID, cyst, ectopic, torsion, TOA), testicular torsion. **LLQ:** diverticulitis, inguinal hernia, renal calc, GYN (menses, PID, cyst, ectopic, ovarian torsion, TOA), testicular torsion, Crohn's disease, colitis. **Epigastric:** GERD, PUD, gastritis, pancreatitis, MI. **Periumbilical:** pancreatitis, SBO, appy, AGE, perforated viscus, nonspecific. **Umbilical pain:** poss appy (tip of appendix may be behind umbilicus). **Suprapubic:** UTI, retention, prostatitis, PID (longer duration of SXS, CMT, and adnexal tenderness), uterine problems. **GU/GYN etiologies,** such as **hernia** or **ovarian torsion,** must also be considered and ruled out

(cont.)

ABDOMINAL PAIN (cont.)

MANAGEMENT

- Consider age, pain severity, hemodynamic stability, risk for serious etiology
- **High risk:** NPO, IV NS, analgesia (see "Pain")
  - Antiemetic, CBC, chem panel CRP, LFT/lipase, lactate, venous blood gas if AMS or severe vomiting
  - UA/UCG, FSBS, recheck abd, pain, fluid tolerance, possible GC/chlamydia
  - Imaging: CXR (infiltrate, free air); KUB/abd; RLQ ultz (e.g., appendicitis); RUQ ultz for gallbladder; CT abd/pelvis
  - Surgical consult; Abx anaerobic coverage for sepsis
- **Low risk:** analgesia, antiemetic, dip UA/UCG, FSBS. X-rays not usually indicated for constipation
- **Trauma:** ABCs, O_2, IVs, EKG monitor, pulse ox, gastric tube, urinary cath. Labs: CBC, chem panel, type and cross, lactate level, lipase, UA
  - CXR, FAST exam, CT if stable. Diagnostic peritoneal lavage if unstable. Flat and upright abd x-ray (KUB). Skeletal survey (assess physical abuse). Surgical consultation

DICTATION/DOCUMENTATION

- **General:** level of distress, anxiety. Pt alert and in no acute distress
- **VS and SaO$_2$:** elevated temp, tachypnea, tachycardia
- **Skin:** PWD, no diaphoresis, cyanosis, or pallor
- **Abd:** flat without distension. No surface trauma, scars, incisions. Bowel sounds are present in all four quadrants. No tenderness, guarding, rigidity to palpation. No tenderness, mass, pulsation in epigastric area. No organomegaly. Negative Murphy's sign. No periumbilical tenderness. No rebound in the lower quadrants. No tenderness over McBurney's point. No suprapubic tenderness or distension. Good femoral pulses bilaterally. No hernia noted
- **Back:** No CVAT
- **Extremities:** FROM (include chest, GU, vaginal, rectal, neuro exam as indicated)

⚪ TIPS

- Distraction needed for good exam
- A period of observation and serial reexaminations of abd pain are essential
- Pregnancy test for all females >11 years
- Be wary of very young, pregnant, immunosuppressed
- Take another, thorough look at "bounce-back" pts with abd pain (e.g., recurrent appy)
- Negative ultz/CT does not eliminate Dx of appy
- Hemodynamic instability and severe abd pain = emergent pt; identify surgical abd and obtain early surgical consult
  - Ensure clear aftercare instructions if discharging a child with abdominal pain of unclear etiology and indicate need to return for signs of possible appy that may develop over time

DON'T MISS!

- Left referred shoulder pain (Kehr's sign)
- Periumbilical ecchymosis (Cullen's sign)
- Flank ecchymosis (Grey Turner's sign)
- Child maltreatment—blunt abdominal trauma

VOMITING AND DIARRHEA

HX
- Changes in appearance and behavior
- Fussy, restless, irritable, weak, lethargic
- F/C
- N/V, appetite, fluid intake, tolerating PO, wet diapers, BM, constipation, frequency of feeding, level of thirst
- Vomiting: number of episodes, bilious, blood, posttussive. Diarrhea: number of episodes, watery, blood, "currant jelly," mucus, pus
- Recent URI, cough, viral illness
- Abd pain; groin, testicular, back pain
- Urgency, frequency, dysuria; increased or decreased urination
- Sick contacts, recent travel
- LNMP, vaginal bleeding or discharge, sexually active
- Meds: recent Abx use (*C. diff*)
- Allergies/immunizations

PE
- **General:** alert, active, fussy, withdrawn, weak, irritable, lethargic
- **VS and SaO$_2$:** fever, tachycardia, hypotension
- **Skin:** PWD; cap refill, pale, cool, moist; jaundice, poor turgor, tenting of skin (skin pinch returns slowly) pallor, cyanosis, mottling
- **HEENT:**
  - **Head:** normocephalic
  - **Eyes:** sclera and conjunctiva normal, moist and bright, tears, PERRLA, EOMI; sunken, dry, dull
  - **Ears:** canals and TMs clear
  - **Nose:** patent, rhinorrhea
  - **Mouth/Throat:** MMM, normal intraoral moisture, posterior pharynx clear, erythema, exudate, lesions
- **Neck:** supple, lymphadenopathy, meningismus, FROM
- **Chest:** accessory muscle use, retractions, CTA bilaterally, crackles, rhonchi, or wheezing
- **Heart:** RRR, normal tones, no murmurs, rubs, or gallops
- **Abd:** flat, round, distended. Surface trauma or scars. BSA auscultated. Guarding, rebound (jump up and down), response to heel tap, rigid, tenderness, masses, hepatosplenomegaly. Rebound or tenderness over McBurney's point. Suprapubic fullness or distention
- **GU: Male:** normal external genitalia, foreskin, urinary meatus, hernia, rash, femoral pulses. Testicular pain, swelling, position; cremasteric reflex. **Female:** discharge, CMT, os closed, adnexal fullness or TTP
- **Rectal:** blood, pain, mass, fecal impaction, tumor
- **Back:** CVAT, ecchymosis
- **Extremities:** FROM, tenderness, distal motor neurovascularly intact
- **Neuro:** alertness, GCS 15, no focal neuro deficits

(cont.)

VOMITING AND DIARRHEA (cont.)

MDM/DDx

Early identification of pts with **dehydration** or **potentially life-threatening causes of V/D** should be the first priority. Normal temperature, hemodynamic stability, and lack of serious comorbidities are reassuring findings. In spite of many specific etiologies for V/D, most children are discharged home with a nonspecific diagnosis. V/D in children is often caused by benign and self-limiting causes such as **AGE** or **mesenteric lymphadenitis**. Norovirus remains by far the most common cause of AGE in children. In younger infants with vomiting, consider **pyloric stenosis**. Peak incidence for **intussusception** is 6 to 12 months; child often presents with lethargy and pain that comes in "waves." Infants may also experience milk or **formula intolerance, lactose intolerance, or GERD.** Colicky abd pain may be caused by **renal calculi** or **hepatobiliary causes.** Signs of acute UTI may be subtle or absent; abd pain is often the only complaint. **Colic, AGE,** and **constipation** are diagnoses of exclusion after a thorough investigation rules out more serious etiologies. **GYN etiologies,** such as **ovarian torsion** or **ectopic pregnancy,** must be considered and ruled out. A complaint of similar pain with new progression should prompt consideration of **ovarian cyst, STI, and PID.** Diagnosis of **serious surgical problems,** such as **appendicitis, intussusception, volvulus, strangulated** or **incarcerated hernia,** or **testicular torsion,** is vital. **Sudden** or **progressive abd pain, uncontrolled V/D, unstable vital signs,** or **altered mental status** in any child are indications for hospital admission. It is important to consider **extra-abd causes** of abd pain in children, especially if preverbal. Neurological problems that cause vomiting include occult **head injury** or **tumor.** Pulmonary symptoms with tachypnea and hypoxia should prompt investigation of **PE** or **pneumonia.** Metabolic problems like **DKA** can present with vague, diffuse abd pain and vomiting. Underlying inflammatory etiologies, such as **SLE** or **HSP,** are often associated with complaints of abd pain. Also consider **sickle cell crisis, ETOH, toxins, medications,** or **OD.** Psychogenic reasons include **anorexia, bulimia,** or **depression.** Intractable or cyclical vomiting: **cannabinoid hyperemesis syndrome**

(cont.)

VOMITING AND DIARRHEA (cont.)

MANAGEMENT

Labs

- FSBS; no other specific studies are indicated for an afebrile child with mild to moderate dehydration who is tolerating oral fluids
- If concern for severe dehydration or underlying illness: CBC with diff, chem panel, UA/UCG; possible LFTs/lipase. Possible urine and blood cultures, LP
- Stool analysis: WBC and culture may be helpful if concern for dysentery; *C. difficile* toxins if >12 months and recent Abx; stool for O&P if watery diarrhea > 14 days; or travel to an endemic area

Imaging

- CXR if respiratory symptoms present and concern for pneumonia
- Ultz and CT not generally indicated unless concern for appendicitis or other intra-abd etiology

Rehydration

- Oral rehydration with ORS is treatment of choice for children with mild to moderate dehydration
- Vomiting: offer 1 tsp ORS every 5 minutes; wait 10 minutes if vomiting and repeat
- Diarrhea: offer 1/4- to 1/2-cup fluids every time child has diarrhea stool using Pedialyte, rehydralyte, or infalyte
- Homemade solution: 1 quart of water + 1/2 to 1 tsp salt + 6 to 8 tsp sugar + 1/2 tsp of baking soda (can add 1/2–1 cup unsweetened orange juice, coconut water, or mashed banana)
- Breast milk, rice water, and diluted cooked cereals are helpful for diarrhea
- IV rehydration: NS 20 mL/kg over 10 to 15 minutes if unable to tolerate oral fluids. Repeat IV bolus until HR, cap refill, UOP, LOC normal
- Maintenance fluids for 24-hour period: <10 kg: 100 mL/kg over 24 hours; 10 to 20 kg: 1,000 mL + 50 mL for each kg more than 10 kg over 24 hours; >20 kg: 1,500 mL + 20 mL for each kg more than 20 kg over 24 hours

Meds

- Ondansetron (Zofran): <8 kg 0.15 mg/kg (oral solution of 4 mg/5 mL), PO/ODT, or IV; 8 to 15 kg = 2 mg; 5 to 30 kg = 4 mg; >30 kg = 8 mg
- Antipyretics and antiemetics as needed
- Antidiarrheals in children not usually indicated
- Abx if underlying infection
- Metronidazole for *C. difficile* and *Giardia*
- Tetracycline or doxycycline for cholera if >8 years
- Zinc for growth and development if <5 years in developing countries
- Probiotics
- RotaTeq vaccine for prevention of rotavirus gastroenteritis

(cont.)

VOMITING AND DIARRHEA (cont.)

DICTATION/DOCUMENTATION

- **General:** awake and alert, in no obvious distress. Not toxic appearing, no lethargy
- **VS and SaO$_2$:** afebrile, tachycardia, tachypnea, hypotension
- **Skin:** PWD, normal texture and turgor, no cyanosis or pallor, appears well hydrated, no tenting; no rash
- **HEENT:**
  - **Head:** normocephalic
  - **Eyes:** moist and bright. PERRLA, EOMI, sclera, and conjunctiva clear. Not sunken
  - **Ears:** canals and TMs normal
  - **Nose:** patent
  - **Mouth/Throat:** MMM, posterior pharynx clear
- **Neck:** supple, no meningismus or lymphadenopathy
- **Chest:** no tachypnea or dyspnea noted; no retractions or accessory muscle use. Lungs clear bilaterally, no wheezes, rhonchi, crackles
- **Heart:** RRR, no murmur, gallop, rub; tones clear
- **Abd:** flat, no distention, soft, BSA, NT, no epigastric tenderness, mass. No rebound or tenderness over McBurney's point
- **GU:** wet diaper, normal external genitalia, no rash or hernia. Normal femoral pulses
- **Rectal/Pelvic:** include if done
- **Back:** no CVAT
- **Extremities:** no swelling, edema, tenderness
- **Neuro:** alert, GCS 15, no focal neuro deficits

◆ TIPS

- A period of observation and serial reexaminations of abd pain are essential
- Colic, AGE, and constipation are diagnoses of exclusion

DON'T MISS!

- Dehydration: restless, irritable, lethargic, sunken eyes, poor fluid intake, tenting
- Pregnancy test for all females >11 years
- Hemodynamic instability and severe dehydration = emergent pt
- Signs of surgical abd
- "Bounce-back" pts with abd pain (e.g., appy)
- Lethargy out of proportion to illness (intussusception)

FOREIGN BODY INGESTION

HX

- Most FB ingestions are asymptomatic and a careful history is essential
- Peak incidence 6 months to 4 years
- Child/parent/caregiver reported or witnessed ingestion
- Gagging, coughing, choking, vomiting, or new-onset wheezing with unclear etiology
- FB noted in stool is less common
- FB: coin, pins, screw, toy, button battery (most toxic)
- **Esophageal:**
    - AMS, drooling, gagging, stridor
    - Sore throat, painful swallowing, FB sensation
    - Cough, wheezing
    - Food refusal, vomiting, blood in emesis, weight loss
    - Chest pain
    - Unexplained fever
- **Stomach/lower GI tract:**
    - Abd pain, distension
    - Vomiting
    - Blood in stool
    - Unexplained fever

PE

- **General:** WDWN, level of activity and interaction, distress. Strong cry, playful, withdrawn, irritable, lethargic.
- **VS and SaO$_2$:** tachycardia, tachypnea, hypoxia
- **Skin:** PWD, pallor, cyanosis
- **HEENT:**
    - **Head:** normocephalic, atraumatic
    - **Eyes:** sclera and conjunctiva normal, PERRL, EOMI
    - **Ears:** canals and TMs normal
    - **Nose:** rhinorrhea or nasal flaring
    - **Mouth/Throat:** MMM; secretions, drooling, or stridor. Posterior pharynx clear or swelling, blood noted. Able to swallow, voice normal.
- **Neck:** supple, FROM
- **Chest:** retractions, accessory muscle use, grunting, stridor. Lungs CTA; wheezes, crackles, or rhonchi
- **Heart:** RRR, no murmur, rub, or gallop; tones clear
- **Abd:** soft, BSA, distended, tenderness, masses
- **GU:** normal external genitalia, no lesion, rash, erythema
- **Back:** spinal or CVA tenderness
- **Extremities:** FROM, strength and tone, neurovascular intact
- **Neuro:** alert, active, GCS 15, no focal neuro findings

(cont.)

FOREIGN BODY INGESTION (cont.)

MDM/DDx

The orientation of a coin on an AP view CXR will usually determine whether it is lodged in the esophagus or trachea. Swallowed coins in the esophagus appear round and flat. Coins aspirated through the vocal cords into the trachea have an "on-end" appearance showing only the rim of the coin. Evaluate carefully to be sure the edge is smooth like a coin and not a "step-off" edge like a button battery. Younger children and infants who put objects in their mouths and have poorer control of the oropharynx are at greater risk for FB ingestion; peak age 2 to 3 years. Most **FBs** (coins) are found to be already in the stomach and pass harmlessly in the stool without complications. Pediatric esophageal FBs often get impacted at the upper esophageal sphincter and less commonly at the lower esophageal sphincter (LES) at the gastroesophageal junction. Pointed objects >6 cm long or >2 cm wide can become impaled and caught anywhere in the esophagus. FBs that have passed into the stomach rarely cause problems and are passed easily. However, FBs may become lodged between the small and large intestine at the ileocecal valve. **Retained esophageal FBs** may cause GI mucosal erosion, abrasion, local scarring, or perforation. **Button batteries** in the esophagus are emergent and can cause dangerous mucosal injury and bleeding within 1 to 2 hours. Swallowed **magnets** in the intestines may strongly attract other swallowed magnets or metallic objects through mucosal tissues, leading to **ulceration, pressure necrosis, fistula creation,** or **perforation**. A swallowed combination of magnets and button batteries is especially dangerous. Consider aspirated FB with pneumonia on CXR that does not respond to Abx. Other complications include **GI bleeding, perforation**, or **obstruction**. Rarely, FBs migrate into the aorta, leading to an **aortoenteric fistula** (high mortality), **mediastinitis**, or **peritonitis**

MANAGEMENT

ABCs—SUCTION IF DROOLING

- ▓ **Imaging:** indicated if any history of possible ingestion
  - ▓ "Baby gram": single frontal x-ray including neck, chest, and entire abd usually sufficient to locate object. Most FBs are radiopaque; fish bones, plastic, and wood objects are often not radiopaque. If an object is seen below the diaphragm, further imaging is generally unnecessary unless the patient has previous GI disorders or congenital abnormalities. Radiolucent objects in the esophagus may be better visualized by repeating the study after having the child drink a small amount of dilute contrast.
    Hold contrast if urgent endoscopy is planned; take special care if there are esophageal obstructions or perforation concerns
  - ▓ Ultz or CT or oral contrast if nonradiopaque object suspected
  - ▓ CT/MRI rarely indicated unless esophageal perforation
- ▓ **Endoscopy:** indicated for sharp or long objects, disk batteries, magnets, HX esophageal FB >24 hours. Maintain NPO.
  - ▓ Preprocedure film to verify the presence and location of FB, which may have passed into stomach while waiting. Procedural sedation or general anesthesia required.
- ▓ **Consult:** GI, surgeon, or psych as needed, or social service if maltreatment
- ▓ **Observation** may be appropriate if FB <5 cm and not sharp, nor a magnet or button battery. Repeat x-ray in 8 to 16 hours.

(cont.)

FOREIGN BODY INGESTION (cont.)

DICTATION/DOCUMENTATION

- **General:** WDWN, alert and active child in no acute distress. Not toxic appearing and in no obvious respiratory distress
- **VS and SaO$_2$:** afebrile, no tachycardia or tachypnea, no hypoxia
- **Skin:** PWD, no pallor or cyanosis
- **HEENT:**
  - **Head:** normocephalic, fontanel normal
  - **Eyes:** PERRLA, EOMI
  - **Ears:** canals and TMs normal
  - **Mouth/Throat:** MMM, no secretions, drooling, stridor. Voice normal. Intraoral lesions, posterior pharynx clear, no FB.
- **Neck:** supple, NT, FROM
- **Chest:** no retractions, accessory muscle use, grunting, stridor. Lungs are clear to auscultation. No wheezes, crackles, rhonchi
- **Heart:** RRR, no murmurs, rubs, or gallops; tones clear
- **Abd:** BSA, soft, NT, no distention, masses
- **Extremities:** FROM, strength and tone, neurovascularly intact
- **Neuro:** alert, active, GCS 15, no focal neuro findings

◉ TIPS

- High index of suspicion based on history because most are asymptomatic and tolerating fluids
- Avoid risk of aspiration by inducing vomiting; laxatives rarely used

DON'T MISS!

- Maltreatment: FBs given intentionally to children by abusive parents/caregivers
- Psychiatric disorder: especially teens who ingest substances and perform risk-taking behaviors as a cry for help
- Toothbrush ingestions and bulimia in teenage girls

GENITOURINARY PAIN

HX

- Age of pt
- Onset, intensity, timing, severity, pattern, location
- Lower abd pain, flank pain, groin pain, or urinary meatus pain
- Dysuria, urgency, frequency, difficulty voiding, urinary retention, enuresis, hematuria, F/C
- N/V, constipation/diarrhea, bowel changes, blood in stool
- Appetite, fluid intake, wet diapers
- Fatigue, malaise, arthralgia, myalgia
- Sexually active/STI, HX HIV
- Suspicion or disclosure of sexual abuse/maltreatment
- Toilet trained, toileting habits, and perineal hygiene (independent vs. assisted)
- Recent illness (e.g., mumps, renal calculi, or infection)
- Trauma, sports injuries, assault, MVC, straddle injury; do not confuse mild trauma with testicular torsion
- **Male:** penile/scrotal pain or STS; feels heaviness in scrotum or palp mass; testicular pain, swelling, change in size of testicle(s), penile discharge. Torsion testicle pain usually acute, may radiate to groin or abd or present only as abd pain; HX of similar pain common; onset during sleep; N/V common (60%–70%), peak age incidence neonates and puberty
- **Female:** vulvar/vaginal/perineal pain or STS; vaginal bleeding, discharge, pelvic pain, LNMP, pregnant/EDC, OB HX

PE

- **General:** level of distress
- **VS and SaO$_2$:** fever, tachycardia
- **Skin:** PWD or pale, cool, moist
- **Chest:** resp unlabored, CTA, normal TV
- **Abd:** abrasions, ecchymosis, surface trauma, or distention. BSA, soft, TTP, rigid, guarding, rebound, masses. No HSM
- **Back:** no spinal or CVAT
- **GU:**
  - **Female:** normal external genitalia of young female. Vulvar or labial STS, erythema, excoriation, trauma, vesicles. Labia and urinary meatus. Vaginal opening clear, swollen, discharge. SMR, hymen, CMT, os closed, adnexal fullness, or tenderness. **Rectal:** blood, pain, mass (fecal impaction, tumor, abscess). Inguinal lymphadenopathy, hernia.
  - **Male:** normal external genitalia or circumcised or uncircumcised male. Penile ulcers, papules, discharge, piercing, tattoos. Scrotum normal size, erythema, warmth, STS, lesion, surface trauma. TTP over epididymis, palp "bag of worms" (varicocele). Scrotal abscess, cellulitis, necrosis. Transillumination (hydrocele). Testes normal size, swollen, tender, normal lie, or horizontal/high riding. Cremasteric reflex (normal elevation of testis when inner thigh stroked; present in majority of males between 3 and 12 years). Prehn's sign, which is an elevation of the testicle, relieves pain in epididymitis, not in torsion. "Blue dot sign" may be seen through thin scrotal skin and indicates torsion of the appendage of the epididymis rather than testis, which may retain adequate blood flow on ultz. Inguinal canal: lymphadenopathy, hernia. Inguinal lymphadenopathy, hernia. Hair tourniquet. **Rectal:** blood, pain, mass (fecal impaction, tumor, abscess). Inguinal lymphadenopathy, hernia.

(cont.)

GENITOURINARY PAIN (cont.)

MDM/DDx

The history must correlate with physical findings to rule out sexual abuse. **UTIs** are a common problem in children. Although children with **pyelonephritis** tend to present with fever, it can be difficult on clinical grounds to distinguish **cystitis** from pyelonephritis, particularly in children <2 years. In neonates symptoms include fever, feeding difficulties, irritability, hypothermia, fever, and signs of sepsis. Infants and children up to 3 years may present with fever, irritability, vomiting, and abd pain. Verbal children >3 years may complain of dysuria, abd, or back pain. Caregivers report frequency, enuresis, fever, hematuria, or malodorous cloudy urine. **Balanoposthitis** is an inflammation of the glans and foreskin that causes itching, irritation and pain, penile discharge, groin rash, and dysuria. More common in uncircumcised children, it is often caused by a fungal infection. In infants, penile inflammation may be the cause of excessive crying. **Posthitis** involves only foreskin. **Phimosis**, an inability to retract the foreskin, may also occur in uncircumcised prepubertal males with balanoposthitis. **Paraphimosis** is a urologic emergency that exists when a retracted foreskin is trapped behind the glans penis and is unable to be pulled into the normal position; impaired blood flow can lead to necrosis. **Genital trauma in males** can involve the penis, scrotum, urethra, or bladder. **In females, genital trauma** can involve the vulva, vagina, bladder, or urethra (rare). Consider genitourinary injury with a history of blunt (straddle injuries, pelvic fractures) or penetrating trauma. Assess for blood at the meatus, hematuria, difficulty or inability to void, perineal or periurethral edema, and ecchymosis. Most vaginal injuries are superficial and limited to the mucosal and submucosal tissues. **Urinary retention** is uncommon in children but may be caused by UTI or constipation. Careful investigation of excessive crying in infants and toddlers with an otherwise normal exam should prompt consideration of a **hair tourniquet** on the external genitalia. Any complaint of **testicular pain** should prompt immediate consideration of **testicular torsion**, which is a true urologic emergency that can result in loss of a testicle. Torsion can occur at any age but mostly occurs between 12 and 18 years. Classic presentation is severe testicular or scrotal pain <12 hours duration, inguinal or lower abd pain, and N/V; testis high and horizontal position. Normal cremasteric reflex is usually absent. Consider intermittent testicular torsion with history of sudden, acute, and intermittent sharp testicular pain and scrotal swelling that resolves in seconds to minutes. **Epididymitis** in older adolescents is often related to STI organisms (chlamydia, GC); in younger boys consider structural abnormality. Pain is usually gradual and associated with swelling isolated to the epididymis, although it may extend to the testis. Dysuria, frequency, urethral discharge, and fever may be present. Although the testis is erythematous and edematous, the normal vertical position is maintained as compared to testicular torsion. **Testicular trauma** can cause a hematocele (hematoma in the tunica vaginalis), intratesticular hematoma, or testicular rupture. **Incarcerated inguinal hernia** into the scrotum can present with pain and a scrotal mass, and BSA is heard in the scrotum. **Orchitis** can be viral (mumps, rubella, coxsackie, echovirus, lymphocytic choriomeningitis virus, parvovirus) or bacterial (brucellosis); scrotal skin is erythematous and shiny; and pain moderate to severe. **Epididymo-orchitis** is an inflammation of epididymis that involves the testicle. Consider other etiologies of testicular pain that cause referred pain such as retrocecal appendicitis, urolithiasis, LS spine nerve root impingement, and malignancy. Any isolated painless indurated area or mass should be evaluated for **testicular tumor.**

(cont.)

GENITOURINARY PAIN (cont.)

MANAGEMENT

- **Labs:** UA and urine C&S, CBC with differential, chem panel. Poss BC, urine NAAT for GC/chlamydia. C&S urethral discharge or vagina/cervix.
- **Imaging:** retrograde urethrography and cystoscopy to evaluate trauma. Color Doppler ults, CT scan

UTI

- Most infants >2 months can be safely managed as outpts with close follow-up. Indications for hospitalization and/or IV antibiotic therapy: age <2 months, clinical urosepsis (e.g., toxic appearance, hypotension, poor capillary refill), immunocompromised, vomiting, or inability to tolerate oral medication, lack of adequate outpt follow-up, failure to respond to outpt therapy
- Uncomplicated well, afebrile child without GU abnormalities: treat for 3 to 5 days with third generation cephalosporin or amoxicillin-clavulanate 50 mg/kg/d divided TID. Options include cefixime 16 mg/kg PO × 1 then 8 mg/kg PO daily; cefdinir 14 mg/kg PO daily: ceftibuten 9 mg/kg PO daily. If PCN or cephalosporin allergy: use TMP/SMX (8 mg/kg/d divided Q12h). Complicated or febrile children should be treated for 10 days. May use Pyridium 4 mg/kg TID × 2 days in 6 to 12 years for dysuria
- **Pyelonephritis:** admit for IV Abx: ampicillin and gentamicin, gentamicin alone, or a third or fourth generation cephalosporin
- **Balanoposthitis:** catheterize if unable to void, peds urology consult. Sitz baths, proper hygiene, avoidance of irritants. Candida suspected: clotrimazole 1%, miconazole 2%, or nystatin. Topical Abx ointment BID may reduce dysuria and prevent secondary bacterial balanoposthitis
- **Phimosis:** confirm ability to void; urology referral
- **Paraphimosis:** analgesia, ice, topical anesthetic gel; gentle manual compression of glans penis for several minutes until able to replace foreskin over the glans. Emergent urology consult if unable to manually decompress
- **Epididymitis/Orchitis:** STI suspected: rocephin 250 mg IM *plus* doxycycline 100 mg BID × 10 days or azithromycin 1,000 mg in a single dose. Low suspicion

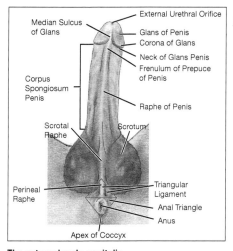

The external male genitalia

(cont.)

GENITOURINARY PAIN (cont.)

for STI trimethoprim–sulfamethoxazole 3 to 6 mg/kg PO Q12h for 10 days **or** amoxicillin–clavulanate 15 to 20 mg/kg PO Q12h for 10 days. Admit if signs of toxicity

- **Torsion:** analgesics, antiemetics, elevate scrotum, NPO. Immediate color Doppler ultz to confirm blood flow and testicular torsion versus torsion of the appendages. Manual detorsion recommended if approaching 6 hours since onset of pain. Definitive treatment is surgery; best salvage rate <6 hours
- **GU trauma:** ice, elevation, and support for hematomas or ecchymoses of penile shaft and scrotum; evaluate injury to testes. Superficial scrotal and penile lacerations can usually be repaired with absorbable sutures. Most vulvar hematomas resolve spontaneously; ice, rest. Ensure ability to void and watch for expanding hematomas that may obstruct the urethra; catheterize if needed. Avoid suture repair of vulvar lacerations if possible. **Vaginal injuries:** ice, analgesia, observe; consult GYN for uncontrolled bleeding
- **Urinary retention:** bladder catheterization, evaluate for constipation, urology consult
- HIV postexposure prophylaxis (PEP)
  - PEP must be started within 72 hours after a recent possible exposure to HIV
  - Basic PEP 2-drug regimen: tenofovir plus emtricitabine QID or BID is preferred; or zidovudine *plus* lamivudine, zidovudine *plus* emtricitabine, or tenofovir *plus* lamivudine. Other alternative regimens may be used per policy
  - Expanded PEP regimen: basic PEP regimen *plus* raltegravir is preferred
- HIV preexposure prophylaxis (PrEP)
  - Indicated for HIV negative adolescents and adults over 35 kg with very high risk of getting HIV through sexual activity or shared IV drug use with a known HIV positive person. Can help provide protection from HIV if pregnant or breastfeeding
- Screen for HIV, liver and renal function
  - Truvada (300 mg tenofovir disoproxil fumarate, 200 mg emtricitabine) daily— stress the importance of adherence to regimen
  - Diagnose and treat other sexually transmitted infections
  - Include counseling regarding regular condom use and sexual risk-reduction strategies in addition to appropriate referral for follow-up and repeat HIV test every 3 months
- Younger teens may be at risk for HIV if they are sexually active young teens, share needles, or are victims of abuse. Also consider transmission risk by accidental exposure to infected human milk, bite wounds, or a puncture wound from a discarded contaminated needle
- *NOTE:* check with infectious disease as regimens may vary
- **STDs:** see www.cdc.gov/std/tg2015/default.htm

DICTATION/DOCUMENTATION

- **General:** level of distress
- **VS and SaO$_2$:** no fever, tachycardia
- **Skin:** PWD
- **Abd:** flat, BSA present, NT to palp
- **Back:** no flank pain or CVAT
- **GU:** normal external genitalia of (un)circumcised male infant/toddler/child/adult. SMR. No inguinal tenderness, lesions, lymphadenopathy. No direct or indirect hernia. Foreskin retracts easily, glans penis normal. Urinary meatus clear without discharge, erythema. Penile shaft without lesions, swelling, tenderness. Scrotum without swelling, erythema, tenderness, induration, crepitus. Testis in normal position, NT. No localized tenderness over upper pole of testis. Transillumination, cremasteric reflex

(cont.)

GENITOURINARY PAIN (cont.)

⊙ TIPS

- Treat sexual partners—STIs
- Pain in testicular torsion is usually acute, but may be insidious
- Testicular torsion: UA neg; WBC: nonspecific leukocytosis (>10 K) in 30%; Doppler ultz diagnostic test of choice (sensitivity 80%–90%)

DON'T MISS!

- Maltreatment: sexual abuse (see "Maltreatment")
- Distinct characteristics of maltreatment:
  - Location of the injury
  - Pattern of the injury
- Correlation of the story to the injury
- Degree or extent of the injury
- History of MOI consistent with age and developmental level of child
- Presence of other unexplained injuries

VAGINAL DISCHARGE

HX

- Onset, intensity, timing, duration
- Characteristics: severity, pattern, and location of pain
- Lower abd pain, F/C, N/V
- Aggravating or relieving factors
- Dysuria, urinary urgency, frequency, hematuria, difficulty voiding, enuresis, urinary retention
- Vaginal bleeding
- Menarche
- Sexually active/STI, LNMP, pregnant/EDC, obstetrical HX, HIV HX
- Suspicion or disclosure of sexual abuse
- Possibility of foreign body insertion
- Toileting habits and perineal hygiene (independent vs. assisted, bubble baths)

PE

- **General:** WDWN, level of distress
- **VS and SaO$_2$**
- **Skin:** PWD
- **HEENT:**
    - **Eyes:** sclera white and conjunctivae pink, injected, tearing, purulence
    - **Mouth/Throat:** MMM, posterior pharynx clear without exudates
- **Chest:** CTA
- **Abd:** BSA, soft, tender, guarding, rebound, rigid
- **Back:** CVAT tenderness
- **GU:** normal external genitalia, SMR, edema, erythema, hematoma, lesions on labia majora, labia minora, urinary meatus, hymen, and clitoris; presence, color, and consistency of discharge, bleeding
- **Pelvic:** CMT, os closed, no adnexal fullness or TTP
- **Rectal:** erythema, edema, lesions, tears, blood, tenderness
- **Extremities:** FROM, good strength and tone bilaterally, neurovascular intact

MDM/DDx

Vaginal complaints in the pediatric population are diverse, and may include nonspecific vulvovaginitis, FB, urethral prolapse, infection, and trauma. **Vulvovaginitis** is the most common GYN complaint in premenarchal girls. Common manifestations include redness, mucoid discharge, soreness, itching, and painful urination. **Candida vaginitis** is characterized by clumped, curd-like white discharge that adheres to the mucosa; most common with recent Abxs, immunosuppressed, or diaper use. **STIs** in children typically result from sexual abuse. Consider GC if green or mucoid vaginal discharge; chlamydia if purulent or mucopurulent discharge (may be present in newborns), or *Trichomonas* if green-yellow and frothy discharge. **FBs** (most often toilet paper) can cause acute and chronic recurrent vulvovaginitis with chronic vaginal discharge, intermittent bleeding, or foul odor. Children with **urethral prolapse** present with bleeding, dysuria, and/or difficulty with urination

(cont.)

VAGINAL DISCHARGE (cont.)

MANAGEMENT

- **Labs:** UA/UCG/Cx; urine NAAT GC/chlamydia; C&S and Gram stain of discharge
- **Vulvovaginitis:** avoid irritants (soap, bubble baths); warm baths, cool compresses to area, emollients, good hygiene measures, avoid wet swimsuits for long periods of time
- **Urethral prolapse:** warm baths, topical estrogen cream twice daily for 2 weeks
- **STIs:** prophylaxis is not routinely recommended for prepubertal victims as the incidence of infections is low after sexual assault in this pt population
    - See www.cdc.gov/std/tg2015/default.htm
- Prepubertal girls have a lower risk of ascending infections but F/U is still required
- **Foreign body removal procedure:** apply a small amount of a topical anesthetic agent to introitus then remove small FBs with a swab or with a warmed irrigation solution

DICTATION/DOCUMENTATION

- **General:** WDWN, alert and active child in no acute distress
- **VS and SaO$_2$:** afebrile, no tachycardia
- **Skin:** PWD
- **Mouth/Throat:** MMM, posterior pharynx clear, no erythema or exudate
- **Abd:** flat, BSA, NT to palp
- **Back:** no CVAT
- **GU:** SMR, normal external genitalia; no edema, erythema, hematoma, lesions on labia majora, labia minora, urinary meatus, hymen, and clitoris; color and consistency of discharge, bleeding
- **Pelvic:** no CMT, os closed, no adnexal fullness or TTP
- **Rectal:** no perirectal erythema, edema, lesions, blood, or tenderness

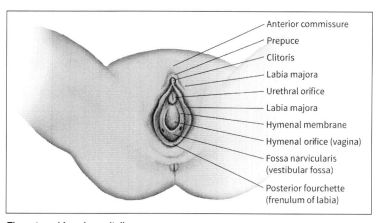

Anterior commissure
Prepuce
Clitoris
Labia majora
Urethral orifice
Labia majora
Hymenal membrane
Hymenal orifice (vagina)
Fossa narvicularis (vestibular fossa)
Posterior fourchette (frenulum of labia)

The external female genitalia

(cont.)

VAGINAL DISCHARGE (cont.)

▶ TIP

■ Larger FBs may need to be removed under procedural sedation/general anesthesia

DON'T MISS!

■ Maltreatment: sexual abuse (see "Maltreatment")
■ Distinct characteristics of maltreatment:
  ■ Location of the injury
  ■ Pattern of the injury
■ Correlation of the story to the injury
■ Degree or extent of the injury
■ History of MOI consistent with age and developmental level of child
■ Presence of other unexplained injuries

FIRST TRIMESTER BLEEDING

HX

- Onset, duration
- OB HX: age of menarche, G, P, TAB, SAB, proof of pregnancy; ABO/Rh
- Clots, cramps, passage of tissue, obvious vag bleed/hemorrhage/discharge, number of pads/hour
- Prenatal care, ultz, B-hCG, previous obstetrical complications, HX HIV
- Abd pain, F/C, N/V, diffuse, lower quadrant, suprapubic
- Urgency, frequency, dysuria, flank or back pain

PE

- **General:** level of distress
- **VS and SaO$_2$**
- **Skin:** cool, pale moist
- **Chest:** tachypnea
- **Heart:** tachycardia
- **Abd:** flat, soft, BSA, NT, no guarding, rebound, rigidity
- **Back:** no CVAT
- **Pelvic:** normal external genitalia, visible bleeding. Vaginal vault is clear, no bleeding, clots, or tissue (if speculum exam done). CMT, cervical os open or closed, uterus nontender and/or normal size, adnexal tenderness or mass (if bimanual done)
- **Rectal:** blood, pain, or mass (fecal impaction, tumor, pelvic abscess)

MDM/DDx

Early bleeding occurs in 25% of all pregnancies, although less frequently in adolescents than older women. About 50% of women who experience bleeding will spontaneously abort (SAB) the products of conception. The majority of SABs are the result of a chromosomal abnormality. Other possible causes are infections, congenital anomalies, endocrine or immunologic disorders, and chemical or radiation exposure. Data collection includes serial B-hCG levels, transvaginal ultz, and baseline ABO type and Rh. In general, pregnant pts with stable VS, FHM on ultz, no adnexal mass, and no sign of acute abd can be discharged home with close F/U. **Ectopic pregnancy** should be suspected in all females with abd pain, vaginal bleeding, B-hCG >1,500 levels, and no gestational sac. Less than half have vaginal bleeding and many have adnexal mass or tenderness. Risk factors for ectopic are IUD use, IVF or infertility, history of ectopic pregnancy, STI, PID, tubal surgery, or smoking. **Urinary tract infections** are common in pregnancy. **Other causes** of lower abd pain in pregnancy that should not be overlooked: **appendicitis, ovarian torsion,** or **tubo-ovarian abscess.**

MANAGEMENT

- Dip UA/UCG, type and Rh, B-hCG
- Possible Hgb/Hct, type and screen, cervical swabs, urine NAAT GC/chlamydia
- Transvaginal ultz and consult as indicated. Close F/U-repeat B-hCG 48 hours
- UTI: send culture and treat (10–14 days) even if asymptomatic
- Nitrofurantoin 100 mg BID; cephalexin 500 mg QID

(cont.)

FIRST TRIMESTER BLEEDING (cont.)

DICTATION/DOCUMENTATION

- **General:** awake and alert in no acute distress
- **VS and SaO$_2$:** no tachycardia or hypotension
- **Skin:** PWD or pale, cool, moist
- **Abd:** flat, BS present in all four quadrants, NT to palpation, no guarding or rebound tenderness
- **Back:** no CVAT
- **Pelvic:** normal external genitalia, no obvious hemorrhage, no blood in vaginal vault; no discharge, no clots or tissue noted, no CMT, no adnexal masses or tenderness, cervical os closed
- **Rectal:** no blood, pain, or mass (fecal impaction, tumor, pelvic abscess)

▶ TIPS

- Ultz guidelines for fetal development
- **~5 weeks:** gestational sac visible
- **5.5 to 6 weeks:** yolk sac visible inside gestational sac (nutrients); "double ring sign" of echogenic chorionic villi and decidua differentiates normal IUP from pseudogestational sac of ectopic pregnancy
- **6 weeks:** fetal pole visible (can measure embryo CRL; may see cardiac flutter)
- **6.5 weeks:** FHM 90 to 110 bpm
- **7 to 8 weeks:** FHM >140 bpm
- B-hCG levels:
  - HCG detectable 12 to 14 days after a +UCG; over 25 is positive for pregnancy; doubles every 2 to 3 days; peaks at 8 to 11 weeks; 5.5 weeks >1,500. Consider ectopic pregnancy with rising B-hCG level and no gestational sac; increased risk in pts with vaginal bleeding, abd pain, and B-hCG HCG >1,500
- RhoGAM indications:
  - If miscarriage or threatened miscarriage occurs within 13 weeks, give 250 IU/50 mcg (minidose) of RhoGAM.

DON'T MISS!

- Significant bleeding, clots, tissue
- Ectopic pregnancy
- UTI or vaginitis
- Rh negative requiring RhoGAM

(cont.)

FIRST TRIMESTER BLEEDING (cont.)

TYPES OF MISCARRIAGES

Threatened	Bleeding <20 weeks; closed cervix, + FHM
Complete	Complete passage of all POC
Incomplete	Passage of some, but not all, POC
Inevitable	Bleeding with dilated cervix
Missed	In-utero death with retention of embryo or fetus <20 weeks
Septic	Incomplete AB with ascending infection of adjacent structures

TERMINOLOGY

Anembryonic pregnancy	Gestational sac >18 mm without yolk sac or embryo (blighted ovum)
Ectopic pregnancy	Pregnancy anywhere outside uterus
Embryonic demise	Embryo >5 mm without cardiac activity (missed AB)
Heterotopic pregnancy	Simultaneous intrauterine and ectopic pregnancy; risk with IVF
Molar pregnancy (hydatidiform mole)	A noncancerous tumor that develops in the uterus as a result of a nonviable pregnancy
Subchorionic hemorrhage	Blood between the chorion and uterine wall seen on ultz

(cont.)

FIRST TRIMESTER BLEEDING (cont.)

ULTRASOUND FINDINGS

No IUP No adnexal mass B-hCG <1,500 clinically stable	Refer to GYN for repeat B-hCG in 48 hours or admit for D&C if hemorrhage or incomplete AB
No IUP No adnexal mass, B-hCG >1,500	Consult GYN for possible ectopic pregnancy
Viable IUP	Refer to GYN for follow-up and prenatal care
Nonviable IUP	Close GYN follow-up for incomplete AB vs. ectopic or admit for hemorrhage
Gestational sac <20 mm or fetal pole > 5 mm and no FHM	Close GYN follow-up for repeat ultz and B-hCG Threatened AB or blighted ovum
Empty sac >20 mm or fetal pole >5 mm and no FHM	Urgent GYN consultation for management of failed pregnancy

Exam: ultz obstetrical <14 weeks complete, transvaginal

Patient age, signs and symptoms (vaginal bleeding, clots, cramps), LNMP or gestational age in weeks. Positive pregnancy test or beta-HCG level

Results: no uterine abnormality identified. Note size and thickness of uterus and if an intrauterine gestational sac is visualized (e.g., 5 weeks, 1 day). Document if each ovary was visualized; evaluate size and if blood flow is normal. Identify presence of adnexal mass or free pelvic fluid

BACK PAIN

HX

- **Medical**:
  - Onset, duration, intensity of pain; exact mechanism such as fall, prolonged sitting/standing, lifting, sports, or injury related
  - Provoking, alleviating factors
  - Prior back problems, prior back pain workup
  - Limitation in ROM/ambulation
  - Quality and radiation of pain
  - Motor or sensory changes, chronic or acute
  - Bowel or bladder retention or incontinence
  - Metastatic disease, weight loss, cough, pain worse at night
  - F/C
  - N/V, abd pain
  - Urgency, frequency, dysuria, hematuria, HX of renal calculi
  - HTN, connective tissue disease (e.g., Marfan's syndrome), obesity, DM
  - SH: smoker, ETOH, IVDA, or illicit drug use
- **Trauma**:
  - Blunt falls, bike injury, MVCs, penetrating trauma
  - Risk factors for maltreatment/interpersonal/family violence
  - See "Maltreatment."

PE

- **General:** level of distress
- **VS and SaO$_2$**
- **Skin:** PWD
- **Chest:** CTA bilaterally; no rales, rhonchi, or wheezing
- **Heart:** RRR, no murmur, gallop rub, clear tones
- **Abd:** soft and NT without masses, guarding, or rebound; BSA, no HSM
- **Back:** note gait to treatment area, symmetric, limp, antalgic, unable to bear weight
  - Surface trauma, soft tissue or muscle tenderness, spasm, mass
  - Point tenderness, step-off, or deformity to palpation at midline
  - CVAT/flank ecchymosis
  - SI notch tenderness, saddle anesthesia, anal wink, rectal tone
  - ROM—flexion/extension/lateral bending and rotation; note whether limited or causes pain
  - SLR—check for radiculopathy: positive sign if radiates below knee
  - Patellar reflexes: brisk, symmetric
  - Muscle strength lower extremities
  - Dorsiflexion/plantar flexion of ankles
  - Heel/toe walk
  - Assess femoral pulses, possible rectal exam
- **Extremities:** status of upper extremity circulation, femoral pulses
- **Neuro:** mental status: affect. LOC, speech; motor: normal gait, muscle strength, and tone for developmental level; CN II–XII intact, DTRs 2+/2+ bilaterally. Meningeal signs

(cont.)

BACK PAIN (cont.)

MDM/DDx

Back pain is uncommon in pediatric pts and the majority of cases are caused by an **acute musculoskeletal injury.** However, severe **trauma** (e.g., MVC with ejection from a vehicle, fall from great height) can also occur. **SCD, idiopathic causes, UTI or pyelonephritis, viral syndromes, or malignancy can also cause back pain**. In the pediatric population, **spondylolisthesis, pars stress reaction, spondylolysis, herniated disk,** and **scoliosis** should be considered. **Chronic pain** may be caused by **developmental problem** (e.g., Scheuermann's kyphosis), **inflammatory spondyloarthropathies**, or **psychological problems**. The main focus is on potential **neurologic emergencies** or other than orthopedic etiology for complaints of pain. **Malignancy:** HX of cancer, recent weight loss, SXS lasting less than 3 months, constant pain at night or at rest. **Infection (discitis, transverse myelitis, epidural abscess**, or **hematoma**): persistent fevers, IVDA, cellulitis, **pneumonia**. Immunosuppression from steroids, transplant, DM, HIV. **Cauda equina syndrome:** bilateral lower extremity pain, weakness, numbness; urinary retention followed by overflow; perineal or perianal anesthesia or poor rectal tone, progressive neurological deficits. **Herniation:** major muscle weakness (strength 3/5 or less), foot drop. **Perforated viscus** may also cause acute back pain.

MANAGEMENT

- Thorough HX and PE to identify possible infectious or malignant etiology or suspected systemic disease
- Consider CBC, ESR, UA, CRP, x-ray if MSK etiology, NSAIDs, TENS, opioids, alternate ice/heat for comfort. Encourage early mobility
- Possible plain L-S spine x-rays
- CT scan if bony pathology suspected; bone scan for spondylolisthesis
- MRI if spinal cord, disc herniation, or soft tissue etiology suspected
- Ortho/neuro referral for pain management, physical therapy, work tolerance evaluation, possible surgical intervention

(cont.)

BACK PAIN (cont.)

DICTATION/DOCUMENTATION

- ▦ **General:** level of distress
- ▦ **VS and SaO$_2$**
- ▦ **Skin:** PWD
- ▦ **Abd:** BSA, NT to palp, no pulsatile masses, good femoral pulses
- ▦ **Back:** able to ambulate to treatment area with/without assistance, or arrived by wheelchair, stretcher, or ambulance. Pt is seated/lying on the stretcher in no obvious/mild/moderate/severe distress. There is no surface trauma. Note abrasions, scars, ecchymosis, or lacerations if recent trauma. No STS or muscle tenderness to palpation, no spasm or mass, and no PT, step-off, or deformity of the bony cervical, thoracic, or LS spine to firm palpation at the midline. No CVA tenderness to percussion, no SI notch tenderness, no saddle anesthesia. ROM—able to stand erect
    - ▦ Normal flexion, extension, lateral bending, and rotation without limitation or complaint of pain. (Note degree of ROM.) Heel and toe walk with good strength
    - ▦ Dorsi and plantar flexion with adequate/diminished strength. Straight leg raises are negative for radiculopathy. Note whether pain is increased in back, buttock, or radiation to what level of leg. Patellar reflexes equal and brisk bilaterally. Good dorsalis pedal pulses and posterior tibial pulse. Sensation to light touch is intact at the great toe web space
- ▦ **Rectal:** (if indicated) normal anal wink or rectal tone
- ▦ **Extremities:** status of upper extremity circulation, femoral pulses
- ▦ **Neuro:** mental status: affect. LOC, speech
- ▦ **Motor:** normal gait, muscle strength and tone for developmental level; CN II–XII intact, DTRs 2+/2+ bilaterally. Meningeal signs.

LUMBAR SPINE X-RAY INTERPRETATION NOTE:

Normal vertebral body and disc spaces. Normal spinal alignment, no evidence of spondylolisthesis. No obvious FX or dislocation. No lytic lesions noted. SI joints appear normal

DON'T MISS!

- ▦ Suspect maltreatment with certain bruising or injuries in various stages of healing or injuries that are not consistent with the MOI. Injuries that are highly specific for maltreatment include pelvic FXs
- ▦ Cauda equina syndrome

(cont.)

BACK PAIN (cont.)

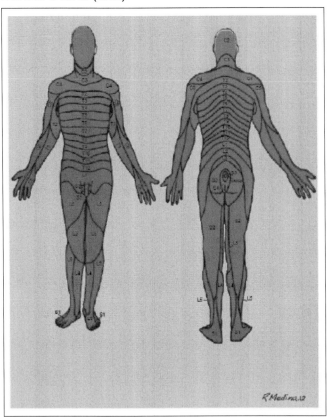

Dermatomes map and locations

(cont.)

BACK PAIN (cont.)

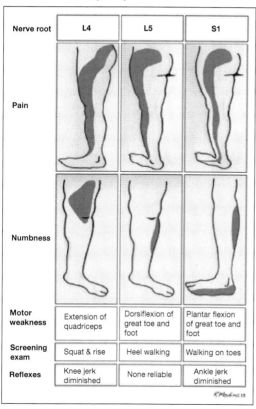

Nerve root	L4	L5	S1
Pain			
Numbness			
Motor weakness	Extension of quadriceps	Dorsiflexion of great toe and foot	Plantar flexion of great toe and foot
Screening exam	Squat & rise	Heel walking	Walking on toes
Reflexes	Knee jerk diminished	None reliable	Ankle jerk diminished

Testing for lumbar nerve root compromise

SHOULDER PAIN

HX

■ Onset, location, duration
■ MOI
■ ROM limitations, pain, F/C
■ Other joints involved
■ Previous shoulder problems
■ Hand dominance, occupation
■ Immunization status
■ Risk factors for maltreatment/interpersonal violence

PE

■ **General:** level of distress
■ **VS and SaO$_2$** (if indicated)
■ **Upper extremity—shoulder**
■ **Note:** compare with unaffected side
■ Obvious deformity/crepitus, shoulder position, rotation (ant/pos dislocation—anterior more common), prominent humeral head. Color, temp, moisture, surface trauma, ecchymosis, open wound, erythema, warmth TTP of clavicle or AC joint, acromion, scapula, humeral head, bicipital groove, STS, muscles—SCM, pectoral, biceps/triceps, deltoid, trapezius, rhomboid, lat. dorsi, rotator cuff quality of pulses; distal neurovascular status
■ ROM: pain or limitation with active/passive movements of abduction/adduction, internal/external rotation
■ Sensation to light touch, sensation over deltoid—axillary nerve injury caused by shoulder dislocation or proximal humerus FX
■ Dorsal hand numbness, weak radial nerve function
■ **Tests:** drop arm, empty can
■ Sulcus sign (test for glenohumeral instability): hold arm straight at side and apply downward traction at elbow. More than 1-cm gap below acromion is positive
■ **Examine:** neck and chest wall for associated injury; evaluate humerus, elbow, wrist, forearm, and hand/fingers

MDM/DDx

Most shoulder injuries in pediatric pts occur as a result of trauma (accidental, maltreatment), overuse, or overtraining ("**Little League shoulder**"). Traumatic shoulder injuries include traumatic **dislocation, proximal humerus FXs, AC joint separation**, and **distal clavicle FXs**. Other causes of pain or instability occur without direct trauma and are seen in swimmers, pitchers, and tennis or volleyball players as a result of **microtrauma, tendonitis, and osteochondritis dissecans (overload = ischemia). Birth injuries,** including FXs or nerve palsy, have also been noted in the neonatal population. Shoulder injuries may be associated with **neurovascular compromise.** Presence of radial and ulnar pulses and capillary refill establishes integrity of peripheral circulation. **Neurologic impairment** is evaluated by motor function such as resisted wrist extension (radial), resisted opposition of thumb (median), and resisted abduction of fingers (ulnar). Motor function includes abduction, rotation, and internal and external rotation. Pts with **anterior shoulder dislocation** (most common) often present with arm slightly abducted, externally rotated, and with loss of deltoid contour. **Posterior dislocation** should be considered in cases of seizures, lightning injuries, or other significant trauma. **FXs of the proximal humerus** or **clavicle** are common findings. Other etiologies are **AC separation, rotator cuff tear, bursitis,** or **tendonitis**

(cont.)

SHOULDER PAIN (cont.)

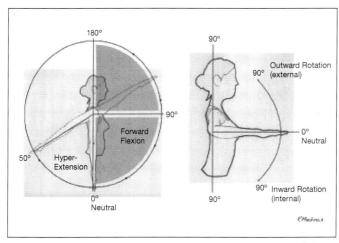

The shoulder range of motion

MANAGEMENT

- Rest, ice, compression, elevation
- (See "Pain") NSAIDs, opioids if needed
- A/P and axial or Y-view x-rays based on MOI
- Urgent reduction of dislocations. Immobilize for comfort with a sling or shoulder immobilizer

DICTATION/DOCUMENTATION

- **General:** level of distress
- **VS and SaO$_2$** (if indicated)
- **Shoulder:** the R/L shoulder is with/without obvious asymmetry or deformity when compared to the R/L shoulder. No surface trauma, ecchymosis, or crepitus. No bony deformity or prominence of the humeral head. No erythema, warmth, or swelling (nontrauma pts). No tenderness to palpation over the clavicle, A-C joint, acromion, scapula, or humeral head. No tenderness to palpation of the bicipital groove or soft tissues. No tenderness to palpation of the muscles of the sternocleidomastoid, pectorals, biceps/triceps, deltoid, trapezius, rhomboid, lat. dorsi, or rotator cuff. No pain or limitation with active or passive abduction/adduction, internal /external rotation, or flexion/extension. Negative "empty can" and "drop arm" test (rotator cuff). No axillary tenderness or lymphadenopathy observed. Normal sensation over the deltoid and ability to flex arm at elbow indicate intact axillary nerve function. Distal motor and neurovascular status is intact

(cont.)

SHOULDER PAIN (cont.)

X-RAY NOTE

For example,, right shoulder series was done to R/O fracture or dislocation. There was no fracture, dislocation, soft tissue swelling, or FB noted

SPLINT NOTE

There was no neurovascular compromise after splint/sling application; the splint was in good alignment and the pt had good sensation and cap refill at the time of discharge

SHOULDER REDUCTION PROCEDURE NOTE

(Adolescent): procedural sedation protocol was followed per institutional protocol and the L/R shoulder was successfully reduced by performing external rotation, Stimson maneuver, scapular manipulation, or traction/counter traction. Neurovascularly intact following procedure; sling and swathe applied after postreduction x-ray demonstrates complete reduction

❯ TIPS

- **AC separation:** pain over joint, possible high-riding bony deformity palp or visible on x-ray
- **Rotator cuff tear:** anterolateral pain referred to deltoid, limited abduction and int rotation; drop arm test, empty can test
- **Bicipital tendonitis:** pain over bicipital groove by shoulder flexion, forearm supination, and/or elbow flexion
- Suspect maltreatment with certain transverse, oblique, and/or spiral FXs; bilateral and/or symmetrical FXs. Epiphyseal separations, bruising, or injuries in various stages of healing or injuries that are not consistent with the MOI. Extremity injuries that are highly specific for maltreatment include metaphyseal–epiphyseal FXs

DON'T MISS!

C-spine injury
- Maltreatment: location/pattern of injury, correlation of story to injury, degree/extent of injury

ELBOW PAIN

HX

- F/C, onset, duration, mechanism of injury (FOOSH)
- Limitation of movement, exacerbation/radiation of pain
- Other joint involvement
- Direct trauma or distraction injury
- Hand dominance, occupation
- Immunization status
- Risk factors for maltreatment/interpersonal/family violence (see "Maltreatment")

PE

- **General:** level of distress
- **VS and SaO$_2$** (if indicated)
- **Upper extremity—elbow**
- **Note:** compare with unaffected side
- Obvious STS, surface trauma, ecchymosis, open wounds, deformity/crepitus, position/ rotation (subluxed radial head—arm held semiflexed, add/pronated), focal erythema, warmth, effusion, joint irritability
- Localize TTP over medial or lateral epicondyle, olecranon, radial head, or distal bicep. Radial/ulnar pulses
- ROM: flex/ext, supin/pron, pain with supination
- Motor/sensory function of ulnar, median, radial nerves
- Distal motor/neurovascular status
- Examine: shoulder, wrist, and hand/fingers

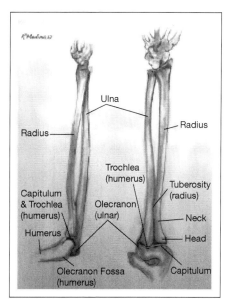

Anatomy of the elbow

(cont.)

ELBOW PAIN (cont.)

MDM/DDx

Children often have minor **strains** or **subluxed radial head (nursemaid's elbow)** but occult **growth plate FXs** must be considered. They are also at a much higher risk for **supracondylar FXs**, which can be associated with significant swelling and **subsequent compartment syndrome**. Elbow dislocations cause severe pain and swelling. A flexed elbow with prominent olecranon suggest a **posterior dislocation;** an extended elbow with shortened upper arm and long-appearing forearm suggests an **anterior dislocation**. A **Monteggia FX** involves the proximal ulna with dislocation of the radial head. **Occult radial head FXs** are common. An elevated **anterior fat pad** or any visible **posterior fat pad** indicates the presence of an FX. Always consider neurovascular compromise. **Clinical suspicion** of FX based on examination requires conservative management with splint and reevaluation. Night stick **FXs**—suspect maltreatment

MANAGEMENT

- Analgesia (e.g., NSAIDs; see "Pain")
- RICE
- X-ray, immobilization with a sling and/or posterior splint; monitor for swelling with supracondylar FX; consult
- Subluxed radial head: no x-ray unless FX concern; manual reduction

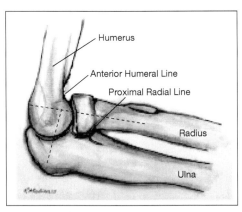

Elbow fracture lines

DICTATION/DOCUMENTATION

- **General:** level of distress
- **VS and SaO$_2$** (if indicated)
- **Elbow:** the R/L elbow is with/without obvious asymmetry or deformity when compared to the R/L elbow. No obvious surface trauma, ecchymosis, or soft tissue swelling is observed. No bony tenderness to palpation of the lateral or medial epicondyle, olecranon, or radial head. No epicondylar or axillary lymphadenopathy. Normal flexion, extension, supination, or pronation. Normal muscle strength. Intact motor and sensation of ulnar, median, and radial nerves

(cont.)

ELBOW PAIN (cont.)

X-RAY NOTE

For example, right elbow series was done to R/O fracture or dislocation. There was no fracture, dislocation, soft tissue swelling, or FB noted. No fat pad elevation seen

SPLINT NOTE

There was no neurovascular compromise after splint/sling application; the splint was in good alignment and the pt had good sensation and capillary refill at the time of discharge

REDUCTION OF SUBLUXED RADIAL HEAD NOTE

The pt's L/R arm was grasped at the distal forearm with counter traction at the elbow. Gentle traction was applied and the forearm was **fully supinated** and **flexed**. There was a palpable "pop" over the radial head. After a few minutes, the pt was using the arm normally. There were no complications

OR

The pt's L/R arm was grasped at the distal forearm with counter traction at the elbow. Gentle traction was applied and the forearm was **hyperpronated**. There was a palpable "pop" over the radial head. After a few minutes, the pt was using the arm normally. There were no complications

⊙ TIPS

- Elbow ossification—CRITOL
  - C—Capitellum—age 1
  - R—Radial head—age 3
  - I—Internal epicondyle—age 5
  - T—Trochlea—age 7
  - O—Olecranon—age 9
  - L—Lateral epicondyle—age 11
- **X-ray:** good lateral film is essential; "figure 8" or hourglass sign at distal humerus. Fat pad elevation: anterior "sail sign" or any visible posterior fat pad is abnormal even if no FX seen
- **Anterior humeral line:** should intersect the middle third of the capitellum on lateral view. FXs will often displace the capitellum posteriorly
- **Radio-capitellar line:** a line down the middle of the radius should bisect the capitellum in both AP and lateral view
- **Monteggia FX—dislocation:** mid or proximal ulnar FXs—dislocated radial head
- **Note:** if FXs are intra-articular or bicondylar
- **Document suspected occult FX:** splint or sling for conservative management
- Refer for repeat x-ray in 7 to 10 days
- **Ortho referral:** displaced, unstable, open, or intra-articular FXs; FX >30% radial head; FX >3 mm or 30° displaced

(cont.)

ELBOW PAIN (cont.)

DON'T MISS!

- Peripheral nerve injury
- Upper extremity neurovascular compromise
- Maltreatment: location/pattern of injury, correlation of story to injury, degree/extent of injury. Suspect maltreatment with certain transverse, oblique, and/or spiral FXs; bilateral and/or symmetrical FXs; epiphyseal separations, bruising, or injuries in various stages of healing or injuries that are not consistent with the MOI

WRIST PAIN

HX

- MOI
- Onset, duration of pain, F/C
- Movement limitation
- Occupation; dominant hand
- Immunization status
- Risk factors for maltreatment/interpersonal/family violence (see "Maltreatment")

PE

- **General:** level of distress
- **VS and SaO$_2$** (if indicated)
- **Upper wxtremity—wrist**
- **Note:** compare with unaffected side
- Obvious STS, surface trauma, ecchymosis, open wounds, deformity/crepitus, position, erythema, warmth, focal mass
- Focal TTP or fullness, pain over scaphoid to direct palp or axial load of thumb, pain with radial deviation
- Radial/ulnar pulses
- ROM: flex/ext, ulnar/radial deviation
- Motor/sensory function of ulnar, median, radial nerves
- Distal motor/neurovascular status
- **Examine:** shoulder, elbow, and hand/fingers
- **Motor/Sensory function:** ulnar, radial, median nerves
- **Phalen's or Tinel's sign** (carpal tunnel syndrome)
- **Finkelstein test** (De Quervain's tenosynovitis)

MDM/DDx

Most wrist FXs are **uncomplicated** FXs of the distal radius and/or ulna but can be more serious based on degree of angulation or displacement. FX or **ligamentous injuries** of the carpal bones are uncommon but can lead to loss of mobility and functional impairment. Hyperextension mechanism should prompt evaluation of scaphoid FX, a common and easily missed carpal FX. Most **scaphoid** FXs (usual mechanism of scaphoid injury is a fall onto a dorsiflexed or extended hand) involve the narrow waist of the bone; compromised blood flow to the proximal portion of the bone can lead to avascular necrosis. Assessment of the alignment and lunate–capitate relationship is vital in the consideration of rare but serious **lunate** or **perilunate dislocations**. These injuries are most often associated with a history of extreme flexion or extension of the wrist. Soft tissue injuries, such as **sprains** or **tendonitis**, can also cause prolonged pain or instability. **Carpal tunnel syndrome** results in compressive neuropathy of the median nerve and presents with burning and numbness of the volar surface of the first three digits. May be caused by video games or repetitive movement in sports or musical instruments.

MANAGEMENT

- Analgesia: NSAIDs (see "Pain")
- RICE
- Wrist brace, volar splint, ulnar gutter splint, thumb spica splint
- Conservative splinting and recheck for possible growth plate FX or scaphoid FX

(cont.)

WRIST PAIN (cont.)

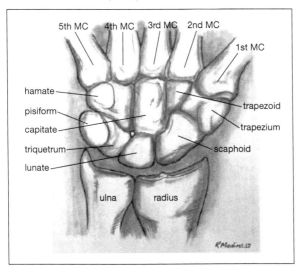

The bones of the wrist

DICTATION/DOCUMENTATION

- ▓ **General:** level of distress
- ▓ **VS and SaO$_2$** (if indicated)
- ▓ **Wrist:** the R/L wrist is with/without obvious asymmetry or deformity when compared to the R/L wrist. No surface trauma, open wounds, swelling, or obvious deformity. No overlying erythema or warmth. No bony crepitus or focal area of TTP. No scaphoid fullness or tenderness to direct palpation or axial load. Normal flex/ext, ulnar/radial deviation. Motor/sensory function of ulnar, radial, median nerves intact. Ulnar and radial pulses intact. Negative Phalen's/Tinel's sign (carpal tunnel syndrome)

X-RAY NOTE

There was no FX, dislocation, soft tissue swelling, or foreign body noted. Normal joint spaces noted

SPLINT NOTE

There was no neurovascular compromise after splint/sling application; the splint was in good alignment and the pt had good sensation and capillary

(cont.)

WRIST PAIN (cont.)

⊃ TIPS

- **Maltreatment:** location/pattern of injury, correlation of story to injury, degree/extent of injury
- Suspect maltreatment with certain transverse, oblique, and/or spiral FXs; bilateral and/or symmetrical FXs. Epiphyseal separations, bruising, or injuries in various stages of healing or injuries that are not consistent with the MOI. Extremity injuries that are highly specific for maltreatment include metaphyseal–epiphyseal FXs

DON'T MISS!

- Navicular/scapular FXs—most commonly injured carpal bone, easily missed, and can lead to avascular necrosis
- Lunate or perilunate dislocations

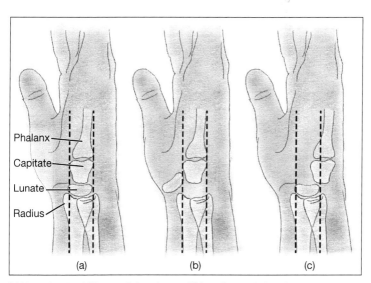

(a) Normal wrist, (b) lunate dislocation, and (c) perilunate dislocation

HAND PAIN

HX

- Medical
  - F/C
  - Recent illness
  - Rash
  - Joint pain
- Trauma
  - MOI: work or sports related; hyperextension/flexion, crush, forceful abduction of thumb
  - Time of injury; crush injury, possible FB
  - Animal or human bite
  - High-pressure puncture injury
  - Movement limitations
  - Feeling of fullness, throbbing pain, swelling of fingertip, proximal lymphangitis
  - Occupation; hand dominance
  - Work-related injury
  - Onset, duration, delayed presentation
  - PMH: recent infection/trauma, chronic steroid use, DM, connective tissue disorders
  - Immunization status
  - Risk factors for maltreatment/interpersonal/family violence (see "Maltreatment")

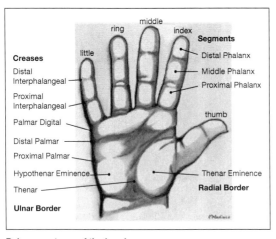

Palmar anatomy of the hand

(cont.)

HAND PAIN (cont.)

PE

- ▪ **General:** level of distress
- ▪ **VS and SaO$_2$** (if indicated)
- ▪ **Upper extremity—hand/fingers**
- ▪ **Note:** compare with unaffected side
- ▪ Color, temperature, ecchymosis, open wound, bleeding, erythema, warmth, exudate, sensation, two-point discrimination
- ▪ Note local or diffuse STS or fusiform swelling of digit
- ▪ TTP, bony step-off, crepitus, or deformity, sensation to light touch
- ▪ Pulses and capillary refill, distal neurovascular status
- ▪ FROM, including isolated FDS/FDP of each digit
- ▪ Normal cascade of fingers, no malrotation (all fingers point toward scaphoid)
- ▪ Examine open wounds under good light with bloodless field; include range of motion and against resistance, and repeat under anesthesia
- ▪ **Flexor tendons:** FDS and FDP
- ▪ **Extensor tendons**
    - ▪ **Abductor pollicis longus and extensor pollicis brevis:** abduct thumb from other fingers
    - ▪ **Extensor carpi radialis longus and extensor carpi radialis brevis:** make fist and extend hand at wrist
    - ▪ **Extensor pollicis longus:** palm down and raise thumb
    - ▪ **Extensor carpi ulnaris:** ulnar deviation intact extension of digits against resistance
    - ▪ **Ligaments:** ulnar collateral ligament of thumb has strong opposition
- ▪ **Nerves**
    - ▪ **Ulnar nerve:** abduct fingers against resistance: sensation on ulnar surface, little finger
    - ▪ **Median nerve:** oppose thumb and little finger: enervates palmar surface of thumb, index, middle, and half of the ring finger
    - ▪ **Radial nerve:** extend wrist and fingers against resistance: sensation on dorsal web space between thumb and index finger
- ▪ **Nails**
    - ▪ Nail avulsion, tissue avulsion, partial/complete amputation, subungual hematoma, nail bed injury
- ▪ Include examination of shoulder, elbow, hand/finger

MDM/DDx

Infections of the fingers and hand include local **paronychia, felon, cellulitis**, and **flexor tenosynovitis**. Soft tissue injuries such as minor sprains are common. More serious injuries involve the volar plate or lateral collateral ligament. Extensor tendon damage can result in permanent deformity such as a **mallet finger** or **Boutonniere deformity**. Strength and function of the FDS and FDP against resistance evaluates the **flexor tendons**. **Bony injuries include fracture or dislocation**: finger dislocations are relatively common pediatric injuries. **Dislocated digits** should be reduced. Injury to the middle phalanx often causes a small avulsion FX or damage to the volar plate. Note swelling and ecchymosis on the volar surface; prompt and concurrent fracture considered. Orthopedic consultation is needed if unable to reduce an FX, **unstable** FXs that involve >25% of the articular surface, **unstable ligamentous injury,** or potential serious **closed space infection** of a finger or hand

(cont.)

HAND PAIN (cont.)

MANANGEMENT

- **Paronychia:** warm soaks, NSAIDs. Use #10 scalpel or blunt instrument to "sweep" and elevate nail fold to promote drainage. Keep open with wick of packing gauze. Hot soaks. Usually no Abx. If severe, Abx selected based on exposure to oral flora resulting from nail biting and finger sucking. Consider felon, herpetic whitlow
- **Felon:** x-ray if concern for osteomyelitis or FB. Digital block and decompress with vertical incision over volar distal phalanx, which is least likely to cause damage and avoid DIP flexor crease. Pack loosely, splint. Abx as for cellulitis or antiviral if herpes suspected (do not I&D)
- **Flexor tenosynovitis:** culture discharge, including fungal, possible CBC, ESR, x-ray. Analgesia, splint in POF. Abx: Vancomycin, Cipro, Rocephin with MRSA coverage. Possible surgical irrigation and drainage of tendon sheath
- **Mallet finger:** analgesia, x-ray, splint PIP joint in full extension for 6 weeks
- **Boutonniere deformity:** analgesia, x-ray, splint PIP joint in full extension for 6 weeks
- **Ulnar collateral ligament injury (gamekeeper's** or **skier's thumb):** thumb spica splint
- **Tendon injuries:** lacerations over a tendon can sometimes be loosely approximated, the hand immobilized, prophylactic Abx given, and referred for surgical repair
- **Distal tuft FXs:** splint with DIP joint in extension; splint should extend past tip of distal phalanx for protection. No need to reduce comminuted tuft FXs; approximate fragments by compression decrease pain and swelling
- **Nail injuries** are commonly associated with distal phalanx FXs. Significant nail bed lacerations are cleaned and repaired using fine (e.g., 6–0) absorbable sutures. If nail plate is displaced from the nail root, clean gently with saline and replace under eponychium—may loosely suture in place
- **Phalanx FXs**: FXs of the neck of the proximal phalanx occur almost exclusively in children; easily missed because of cartilaginous distal FX fragment
- **Metacarpal FXs:** shaft FXs are more common but may be periarticular. Base of thumb most common FX. Rolando FX: comminuted FXs of base of thumb metacarpal caused by hyperextension and hyperabduction. FXs of the distal fourth or fifth metacarpal are common and referred to as "boxer's FX" and are best immobilized in an ulnar gutter splint

DICTATION/DOCUMENTATION

- **General:** level of distress
- **VS and SaO$_2$** (if indicated)
- **Hand/Fingers:** the R/L hand is with/without obvious asymmetry or deformity when compared to the R/L hand. No swelling, erythema, atrophy, or obvious deformity. No surface trauma, open wounds, nail avulsion, tissue avulsion, partial or complete amputation, subungual hematoma, or bony deformity. Normal cascade of fingers. Normal flexion and extension of the fingers. FDS and FDP intact against resistance. No focal fullness, throbbing pain, swelling of fingertip. NT to palpation—describe exact joint, digit, or location. Pulses and cap refill

(cont.)

HAND PAIN (cont.)

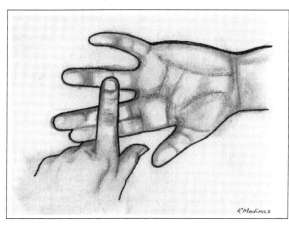

Assessment of flexor digitorum profundus (FDP)
Note: Hold middle phalanx in complete extension and evaluate the strength of flexion of the distal phalanx (DIP). Repeat for each digit.

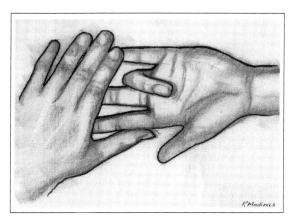

Assessment of flexor digitorum superficialis (FDS)
Note: Hold nonaffected digits in complete extension and evaluate the strength of flexion of the PIP joint with the DIP joints in extension. It is important to eliminate the use of intrinsic palmar muscles in order to isolate the flexor tendon.

(cont.)

HAND PAIN (cont.)

X-RAY NOTE

There was no FX, dislocation, soft tissue swelling, or foreign body noted

SPLINT NOTE

There was no neurovascular compromise after splint application; the splint was in good alignment and the pt had good sensation and capillary refill at the time of discharge

⬤TIP

■ **Maltreatment:** Location/pattern of injury, correlation of story to injury, degree/extent of injury. Suspect maltreatment with certain transverse, oblique, and/or spiral FXs; bilateral and/or symmetrical FXs; epiphyseal separations; bruising and burn; or injuries in various stages of healing; and/or injuries that are not consistent with the MOI. Extremity injuries that are highly specific for maltreatment include metaphyseal-epiphyseal FXs

DON'T MISS!

■ Flexor tendon injuries
■ Vascular injuries
■ Compartment syndrome
■ High-pressure penetration
■ Tenosynovitis

■ Intra-articular FXs or FXs with rotational malalignment
■ Consider **flexor tendon** involvement in any trauma to forearm, palm, or digits

HIP/PELVIC PAIN

HX

- Onset, duration, characteristics, aggravating or alleviating factors, unilateral or bilateral
- MOI: known injury, repetitive mechanism, change in activity, change in athletic sports
- Hear or feel snap or pop; pain related to activities
- Movement/ambulation limitations; morning stiffness
- Ability to bear weight or altered gait
- Caregiver report that child seems well other than refusal to bear weight
- Other joint involvement
- Pain referred to thigh, knee, groin
- Recent F/C, URI, pain at night or night sweats, weight loss
- Back pain, numbness, tingling of lower extremities
- Recent viral illness
- Infants: irritable, poor feeding
- PMH: previous injury or surgery; sickle cell disease, Lyme disease, malignancy; chronic inflammatory joint disease; systemic diseases, such as IBD, psoriatic arthritis, ankylosing spondylitis, or inflammatory rheumatic disease, that are associated with spondyloarthropathy
- Meds: analgesia, steroids
- Immunization status
- Risk factors for maltreatment/interpersonal/family violence (see "Maltreatment")

PE

- **General:** level of distress
- **VS and SaO$_2$:** fever
- **Skin:** PWD, hot, cool, pale, moist
- **Lower extremity—hip**
- **Note:** compare with unaffected side, observe gait, ability to bear weight
- Obvious asymmetry, deformity/crepitus, external rotation shortening, STS, effusion, surface trauma, ecchymosis, open wounds, position, erythema, warmth, focal mass, joint irritability
- TTP over symphysis pubis, ischial bone, iliac crest, trochanter, SI notch, buttocks, quadriceps, femoral triangle, inguinal ligament, inguinal lymphadenopathy, mass
- Femoral pulses, distal neurovascular status
- ROM: flex/ext, abduction/adduct, int/ext rotation. ROM unlimited and without pain
- Normal flexion to chest (135°), extension (30°), abduction (45°), adduction (across midline, internal/external rotation [45°]). FABER to distinguish hip pain from LSpine problem
- Holds hip flexed and abducted for comfort
- Distal motor/neurovascular status
- Evaluate muscle strength and tone using a 5-point scale
- Examine: abd, groin, LSpine, and lower extremity (especially knee)
- **Galeazzi test:** measure the length of the femur with pt on his or her back and his or her legs in adduction with hips and knees, both flexed at 90°. Knees should be in the same location. Short limbs may be a sign of occult FX, dislocation, or developmental dysplasia of the hip
- **Ellis test:** Evaluate the length of the tibia by holding knees and the medial malleoli together, and checking the position of the knee

(cont.)

HIP/PELVIC PAIN (cont.)

MDM/DDx

MDM for child and adolescent hip pain includes common and benign etiologies, such as **muscle strain** or **mild trauma**, in addition to more serious pathology such as **septic joint**. A wide variety of conditions must be considered because many hip problems present with vague or nonspecific symptoms. Most problems can be categorized as infectious, inflammatory, mechanical, or malignant. **Infectious:** severe, localized pain and inability to bear weight, and fever is common. Possible diagnoses include septic arthritis of the hip or sacroiliac joint, osteomyelitis, abscess of the psoas muscle, Lyme disease, appendicitis; infants with a septic hip joint will classically hold the joint in flexion, abduction, and external rotation. **Inflammatory:** usually gradual onset (except transient synovitis, which is acute), possible skin, nails, or eye involvement, in addition to other joints. May be able to bear weight. Consider transient synovitis, systemic arthritis, or spondyloarthropathy, Kawasaki disease. **Mechanical:** sudden or gradual onset of hip pain that may be referred to thigh or knee, exacerbated by activity; no systemic symptoms. Pain may be caused by minor strain or occult injury; femoral stress FX less common. More serious causes are septic joint, AVN (groin pain, limp, passive abduction, and int/ext rotation of leg, 25 to 45 years), and SCFE (10 to 16 years, M > F, obese, referred knee pain, limp, decreased ROM). **Malignancy:** tumor, leukemia. **Other: sickle cell disease** (see "Child With Limp")

MANAGEMENT

- RICE
- NSAIDs, opioids (see "Pain")
- If unable to bear weight—x-ray, splint/crutches, then recheck 1 to 2 days
- **FX:** ortho consult
- **Transient synovitis:** supportive, reassurance, analgesia, evaluate for septic joint or bone infection, close F/U
- **Septic joint:** CBC with diff (elevated WBC ESR: >40), CRP, blood cultures, consult ortho for joint aspiration (80% + Gram stain) and possible surgery. X-ray, ultz, CT/MRI for effusion. IV Abx for several weeks
- **SCFE:** analgesia, immobilize. AP and frog-lateral x-rays of the pelvis or bilateral hips. Check for position of Klein line (line from superior border of femoral neck should pass through part of femoral head and note degree of displacement). Emergent ortho consult
- **AVN:** analgesia, immobilize. AP and frog-lateral x-rays of the pelvis or bilateral hips (high incidence of bilateral). Check for femoral head lucency, sclerosis, or flattening. MRI if negative x-ray but high suspicion; CT less sensitive. Urgent ortho consult
- **Radiology:** x-rays indicated for possible trauma, possible widened joint space with septic joint, tumor, or malignancy, SCFE. Ultz may help identify small effusions associated with septic joint; consider CT or MRI if plain x-rays are negative but high suspicion for serious etiology in symptomatic pts; bone scan can be helpful in osteomyelitis or malignancy
- If unable to bear weight, consider CT/MRI of hip for occult FX
- **TAD:** lower extremity paresis

(cont.)

HIP/PELVIC PAIN (cont.)

DICTATION/DOCUMENTATION

- ▪ **General:** level of distress
- ▪ **VS and SaO$_2$**
- ▪ **Hip:** able to ambulate to treatment area with/without difficulty or assistance, pain, limp, antalgic gait. No surface trauma, ecchymosis. No erythema, warmth. No deformity, crepitus, or obvious asymmetry of the affected leg when compared to other leg. No TTP over symphysis pubis, ischial bone, iliac crest, trochanter, SI notch, buttocks, quadriceps, femoral triangle, inguinal ligament. No inguinal lymphadenopathy. ROM unlimited and without pain. Normal flexion to chest (135°), extension (30°), abduction (45°), adduction (across midline, internal/external rotation [45°]). Distal motor and neurovascular status are intact

X-RAY NOTE

For example, right hip x-ray series was ordered to R/O FX or dislocation. There was no FX, dislocation, soft tissue swelling, or FB noted

SPLINT NOTE

There was no neurovascular compromise after splint application; the splint was in good alignment and the pt had good sensation and capillary refill at the time of discharge

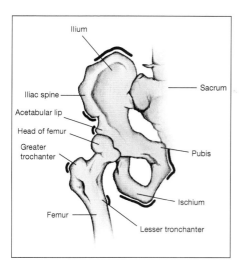

Pediatric hip anatomy

(cont.)

HIP/PELVIC PAIN (cont.)

⊙ TIP

- **Maltreatment:** location/pattern of injury, correlation of story to injury as previously noted, degree/extent of injury. Suspect maltreatment with certain transverse, oblique, and/or spiral FXs; bilateral and/or symmetrical FXs; epiphyseal separations, bruising, or injuries in various stages of healing or injuries that are not consistent with the MOI

DON'T MISS!

- Lower extremity injuries that are highly specific for maltreatment include: metaphyseal–epiphyseal FXs and pelvic FXs

- Septic joint: identify rapidly because of risk of poor blood supply to femoral head
- Intra-abd or pelvic etiology

KNEE PAIN

HX

- Onset, duration, redness, pain, F/C, STS immediate/gradual, ability to bear weight
- MOI—direct trauma, foot planted/knee twisted, valgus versus varus force, falls, jumping from significant height
- Atraumatic knee pain or swelling
- Locking—unable to passively move, 45° flexed (meniscus or cruciate injury); clicking, crepitus, or feeling of giving way (ACL injury)
- Recent illness, fever, loss of appetite, weight loss
- HX patellar or knee joint dislocation/reduction
- Immunization status
- Risk factors for maltreatment/interpersonal/family violence (see "Maltreatment")

PE

- **General:** level of distress
- **VS and SaO$_2$** (if indicated)
- **Lower extremity—knee**
- **Note:** compare with unaffected side, observe gait, ability to bear weight
- Exam often difficult because of pain and swelling. Perform knee exam with pt supine, visualize both legs from the groin to toes and compare. The R/L knee is with/without obvious asymmetry or deformity when compared to the R/L knee
- Obvious crepitus, patella location, STS/effusion, surface trauma, ecchymosis, open wounds, position, erythema, warmth, joint irritability
- TTP over patella, lat/med joint line prox fibula tibial tubercle, popliteal pulse/fullness
- TTP over distal thigh or upper leg (consider infection or malignancy)
- ROM: flex/ext, able to do deep knee bend with symmetry (130°), fully extend knee, internal and external rotation (10°)
- Laxity with valgus or varus stress
- Distal motor/neurovascular status
- **Effusion:** <6 hours with cruciate lig, meniscus, FX. Slower onset and recurrent effusion more likely with meniscus injury. Patella ballottement
- **Tibial sag:** flex 90° and see whether tibia sags posteriorly
- **Lachman/Drawer maneuver**
- **McMurray/Apley compression test**
- *Exam deferred* (McMurray/Apley tests): if pt in significant pain and is unable to perform test, examine: back, hip, ankle, and foot

KNEE X-RAY ORDERING CRITERIA:

- No TTP of knee other than patella
- PT of fibular head
- Inability to flex knee to 90°
- Inability to bear weight (four steps—unable to transfer weight twice onto each lower limb regardless of limping) both immediately and in ED

Source: Adapted from Stiell, I. G., Wells, G. A., Hoag, R. H., Sivilotti, M. L., Cacciotti, R. G., Verbeek, P. R., . . . Michael, J. A. (1997). Implementation of the Ottawa Knee Rule for the use of radiography in acute knee injuries. *Journal of the American Medical Association, 278*(23), 2075–2079. doi:10.1001/jama.1997.03550230051036

(cont.)

KNEE PAIN (cont.)

MDM/DDx

Focus is on differentiating between acute and other (e.g., chronic) conditions that cause pediatric knee pain. **Acute injuries** include **sprain, strain,** or **contusion;** FX or **dislocation. Patellar dislocation** usually occurs laterally and must be distinguished from a **joint dislocation,** which is an orthopedic emergency. External **ligamentous injuries** are more common in adolescents than in pediatric pts and cause pain over lateral ligament and possible laxity of LCL or MCL. **Patellar** or **tibial plateau** FXs may require surgical intervention. Internal derangement injuries usually result in an effusion. **Meniscus tear** usually presents with JLT, pain with weight bearing, +McMurray test, locking, or giving way. ACL injury is associated with immediate severe pain, "popping" sensation, instability, positive Lachman/Drawer test, and inability to ambulate. **PCL tear** is an uncommon injury that results from a fall on a flexed knee or direct trauma to the front of the knee. **Other causes of knee pain** to consider include **prepatellar bursitis** (TTP over patella, swelling and redness over infrapatellar area, and inability to flex or put pressure on knee) and **osteochondritis dissecans** (small fragment of bone and cartilage cracks and loosens because of poor blood supply). There is separation of the bone fragment from the overlying articular cartilage (in pts with open growth plates). These pts C/O generalized knee pain without prior trauma and state that the pain is worse with activity. **Legg–Calve–Perthes Dx** (acute onset of limp, limited hip motion, knee pain; 4–14 years old), **Osgood-Schlatter disease** (pain and STS at site of infrapatellar tendon insertion into tibial tubercle, pain with resisted extension; 9–16 years old, M > F), **septic joint, gout,** or **tumor** may also be issues. In cases of referred pain, think of **SCFE** (see "Child With Limp"). Some children have chronic knee pain caused by **arthritis, tendonitis,** or **patella–femoral syndrome** (vague, anterior knee pain). **Tendonitis** (knee pain exacerbated by going up and down stairs, and prolonged sitting) is common in athletes

MANAGEMENT

- NSAIDs, analgesia
- See "Pain"
- RICE, knee immobilizer, or plaster long-leg splint as indicated
- **Patellar dislocation:** manual reduction for simple horizontal dislocation (lateral most common). Place pt supine, extend knee with gentle, anteromedial pressure over lateral patella to lift patella over femoral condyle
  - Knee immobilizer, crutches
- **Knee dislocation:** assess for vascular injury and immediate reduction; emergent ortho and/or vascular consult
- **Tibial plateau FX:** x-ray, knee immobilizer, crutches with nonweight bearing if FX is nondisplaced or only minimally (4–10 mm) displaced. Surgery needed if open, significantly displaced, or depressed. Consider compartment syndrome

(cont.)

KNEE PAIN (cont.)

DICTATION/DOCUMENTATION

- ■ **General:** level of distress
- ■ **VS and SaO$_2$**
- ■ **Knee:** able to bear weight and ambulate without pain. No surface trauma, STS, or obvious effusion. No overlying erythema or warmth (medical complaints). The R/L knee is with/without obvious asymmetry or deformity when compared to the R/L knee. Pt is able to perform deep knee bend with symmetry (130°), fully extend knee, with internal and external rotation (10°). No tenderness to palpation of the patella, no effusion or ballottement. No tenderness over the infrapatellar tendon (bursitis or Osgood–Schlatter's). No tenderness over the medial or lateral joint line, or the medial or lateral tibial plateaus. No tenderness over the proximal fibular head. No tenderness, fullness, or mass of the popliteal fossa. No quadriceps tenderness. No laxity of the ACL, PCL, MCL, or LCL. May note no collateral ligament laxity to valgus or varus stress. Negative Lachman/Drawer sign. Negative McMurray. Negative Apley compression and/or distraction. Distal motor neurovascular status intact

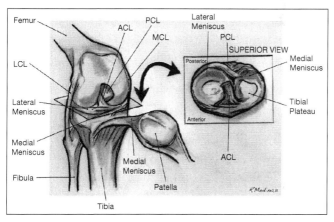

Anatomy of the knee (anterior and superior views)

(cont.)

KNEE PAIN (cont.)

X-RAY NOTE

For example, right knee series was done to R/O fracture or dislocation. There was no FX, no effusion, dislocation, soft tissue swelling, or foreign body noted

SPLINT NOTE

There was no neurovascular compromise after splint/immobilizer application; the splint/immobilizer was in good alignment and the pt had good sensation and capillary refill at the time of discharge

JOINT ASPIRATION PROCEDURE NOTE

The pt was placed in sitting/supine position with knee supported and slightly flexed. The skin was prepped with povidone–iodine solution and cleansed with NS. The site was anesthetized with 1% lidocaine ( ) mL with good anesthesia. The lateral/medial joint space was entered using an 18- or 20-gauge needle. A slight "give" was appreciated as the needle entered the joint capsule. ( ) mL fluid (clear, cloudy, bloody, fat globules) was aspirated. The needle was removed and a dry, sterile antibiotic dressing was placed over the puncture site and a compression dressing (e.g., Ace wrap) was applied. Joint fluid was sent for CBC with diff, glucose, protein, crystals, and C&S. The pt tolerated the procedure well without complication

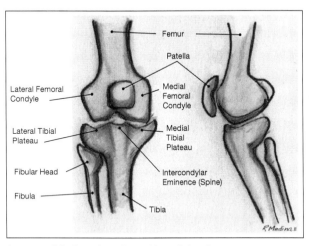

Anatomy of the knee (anterior and lateral views)

(cont.)

KNEE PAIN (cont.)

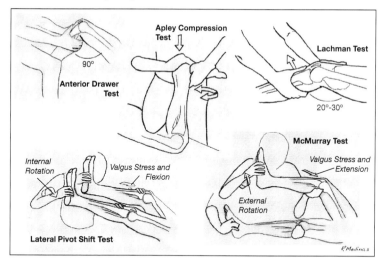

Apley Compression Test

Anterior Drawer Test

90°

Lachman Test

20°-30°

Internal Rotation

Valgus Stress and Flexion

McMurray Test

Valgus Stress and Extension

External Rotation

Lateral Pivot Shift Test

R. Medina.II

Provocative tests of the knee

◗TIP

- **Maltreatment:** Location/pattern of injury, correlation of story to injury, degree/extent of injury (e.g., bruising or injuries in various stages of healing or that are not consistent with the MOI)

DON'T MISS!

- Subtle FXs
- Widened joint space—unstable ligamentous injury
- If joint dislocation—delayed SXS of vascular injury
- Compartment syndrome
- Quadriceps rupture—be sure pt can extend and resist
- Chronic knee pain—pain often worse at night

ANKLE PAIN

HX

- Onset, duration, pain, F/C
- MOI—inversion "rolled," eversion, direct trauma, step from height, "pop" or "snap" at time of injury
- Movement/ambulation, limitations/associated injuries
- Previous ankle injury/surgery
- Recent quinolone use—tendon rupture or worsening myasthenia
- Immunization status
- Risk factors for maltreatment/interpersonal/family violence (see "Maltreatment")

PE

- **General:** level of distress
- **VS and SaO$_2$** (if indicated)
- **Lower extremity—ankle**
- **Note:** compare with unaffected side; observe gait, ability to bear weight
- Obvious asymmetry, deformity/crepitus, STS/effusion, surface trauma, ecchymosis, open wounds, erythema, warmth, dorsalis pedis/posterior tibial pulses; distal neuro-vascular status
- ROM: flex/ext, inversion/eversion
- TTP or deformity over anterior ankle, med/lat malleolus, navicular, proximal fifth metatarsal, calcaneus, Achilles tendon, midfoot/toes
- TTP, STS, ecchymosis over deltoid lig, TFL, PTFL, CFL
- Thompson test—plantar flexion
- Squeeze test—pain along midshaft of fibula when compressed with tibia (high ankle sprain of syndesmosis)
- Talar tilt with valgus/varus stress
- Anterior drawer test
- Peroneal nerve: eversion/plantar flexion
- **Note knee pain:** STS, effusion, pain or deformity over proximal fibula
- Maisonneuve FX: proximal fibular FX with medial malleolar injury
- **Foot and toes:** check proximal fifth metatarsal
- Examine knee (proximal fibula) and foot/toes and evaluate contralateral knee ankle and foot/toes

ANKLE X-RAY ORDERING CRITERIA

- Ankle x-ray: pt at posterior edge or tip of lateral malleolus
- Pt at posterior edge or tip of medial malleolus
- Inability to bear weight both immediately and in the ED
- **Foot x-ray** should be ordered if there is any pain in the midfoot zone and either of the following: pt at base of fifth metatarsal, pt at navicular
- Inability to bear weight both immediately and in the ED

(cont.)

ANKLE PAIN (cont.)

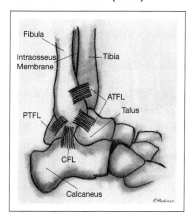

The anatomy of the ankle
Source: Adapted from Stiell, I. G., Greenberg, G. H., McKnight, R. D., Nair, R. C., McDowell, I., Reardon, M., … Maloney, J. (1993). Decision rules for the use of radiography in acute ankle injuries. Refinement and prospective validation. *Journal of the American Medical Association, 269*(9), 1127–1132. doi:10.1001/jama.269.9.1127

MDM/DDx

Ankle injuries most often involve **sprains** caused by an inversion or twisting mechanism that causes pain, ecchymosis, and STS over the ATFL or CFL. Consider **Achilles tendon rupture**, which can present like an ankle sprain. Involvement of the deltoid or medial ligaments should prompt concern for a **Maisonneuve** FX of proximal fibula. **Severe sprains** resulting from complete rupture of the ligament cause immediate marked swelling, ecchymosis, and inability to bear weight and can lead to chronic instability. Point tenderness, deformity, or crepitus over the posterior edge of the medial or lateral malleolus, base of the fifth metatarsal, or midfoot suggest FX. A **distal fibula avulsion** FX is a stable injury. **Bi- or trimalleolar** FXs **and Maisonneuve** FX are unstable injuries requiring urgent orthopedic referral, as do intra-articular and open FXs. Forced dorsiflexion and inversion injuries may cause a **talofibular injury** or **ankle dislocation.** FX **dislocations** of the ankle are rare and are associated with **ruptured ligaments.** These severe injuries are at high risk for **neurovascular compromise** if not reduced immediately

MANAGEMENT

- Analgesia, NSAIDs (see "Pain")
- RICE, if unable to bear weight—crutches, recheck 1 to 2 days
- Air splint, brace, taping. Equine splint for Achilles tendon injury. Splint, crutches, NWB for severe sprain or FX. Gentle ROM, bear weight as tolerated. Orthopedic consult for unstable FX: disruption of mortise, FX/dislocation, bi- or trimalleolar FX

(cont.)

ANKLE PAIN (cont.)

DICTATION/DOCUMENTATION

- **General:** level of distress
- **VS and SaO$_2$**
- **Ankle:** able to bear weight and ambulate without pain. The R/L ankle is with/without obvious asymmetry or deformity when compared to the R/L ankle. Pt can flex/ext, inversion/eversion. No obvious surface trauma, ecchymosis, or STS. No bony TTP over the medial or lateral malleolus
- ATFL, PTFL, CFL NT and without swelling. (May also be referred to generally as medial/deltoid or lateral ligaments.) NT or deformity of the midfoot or over the proximal fifth metatarsal. Good dorsalis pedis and posterior tibial pulses and sensation to light touch normal. Talar tilt test is negative for ligament laxity to valgus or varus stress. Negative anterior drawer. Peroneal nerve is intact with strong eversion and plantar flexion

X-RAY NOTE

For example, right ankle x-ray series was done to R/O FX or dislocation. There was no FX, dislocation, soft tissue swelling, or foreign body noted

SPLINT NOTE

There was no neurovascular compromise after splint application; the splint was in good alignment and the pt had good sensation and capillary refill at the time of discharge

◗TIPS

- **Maltreatment:** Location/pattern of injury, correlation of story to injury, degree/extent of injury. Suspect maltreatment with certain transverse, oblique, and/or spiral FXs; bilateral and/or symmetrical FXs; epiphyseal separations, bruising, or injuries in various stages of healing or injuries that are not consistent with the MOI
- Lower extremity injuries that are highly specific for maltreatment include metaphyseal–epiphyseal FXs

DON'T MISS!

- Salter Harris type-1 FXs with open growth plates
- Peroneal nerve injury (occult injury)
- Achilles tendon rupture
- Check proximal fifth metatarsal or proximal fibular FX

FOOT PAIN

HX

- Onset, duration
- MOI, movement, ability to bear weight
- Ankle or knee pain or associated injuries, soft tissue infection, immunization status
- Risk factors for maltreatment/interpersonal/family violence (see "Maltreatment")

PE

- **General:** level of distress
- **VS and SaO$_2$** (if indicated)
- **Lower extremity—foot/toes**
- **Note:** compare with unaffected side; observe gait, ability to bear weight
- Obvious asymmetry, deformity/crepitus, STS, surface trauma, ecchymosis, open wounds, erythema, warmth, dorsalis pedis/posterior tibial pulses, rash/lesions, open wound, ulcer, plantar wart
- Extensive STS caused by crush injury—consider compartment syndrome
- STS, erythema, exudate, hypertrophy of nail or margins, subungual hematoma
- Hair tourniquet on toes in infants/toddlers
- Distal neurovascular status
- TTP of talus, calcaneus, metatarsals 1 to 5, each MTP joint and IP joint, plantar/dorsal surface
- ROM: plantar/dorsiflexion, inversion/eversion
- Examine: hip, knee, and ankle

ANKLE/FOOT X-RAY ORDERING CRITERIA:

- **Ankle x-ray** should be ordered if malleolar zone pain and any of the following:
  - PT at posterior edge or tip of lateral malleolus
  - PT at posterior edge or tip of medial malleolus
  - Inability to bear weight both immediately and in the ED
- **Foot x-ray** should be ordered if there is any pain in the midfoot zone and any of the following:
  - PT at base of fifth metatarsal
  - PT at navicular
  - Inability to bear weight both immediately and in the ED

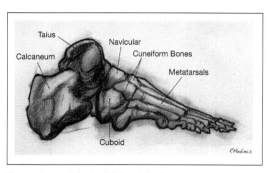

The anatomy of the foot (lateral view)

(cont.)

FOOT PAIN (cont.)

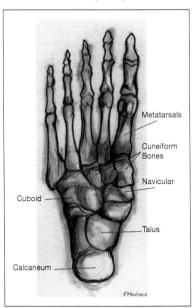

The anatomy of the foot (superior view)
Source: Adapted from Perry, J. J., & Stiell, I. G. (2006). Impact of clinical decision rules on clinical care of traumatic injuries to the foot and ankle, knee, cervical spine, and head. *Injury, 37*(12), 1157–1165. doi:10.1016/j.injury.2006.07.028

MDM/DDx

Injuries with neurovascular deficit, open FXs, **severe crush injury**, or concern for **compartment syndrome** are orthopedic emergencies. Overuse, as well as direct or indirect trauma to the foot, can result in soft tissue injuries, such as **contusions, sprains, or tendonitis**, including plantar fasciitis or bone spurs. Undetected hair tourniquet of a toe is part of the evaluation of unexplained pediatric crying. Bony injuries include FXs or dislocations. Most FXs of the toes and nondisplaced FXs of the metatarsals are not clinically significant. However, intra-articular, displaced, and multiple metatarsal FXs require prompt referral. Midfoot injuries should be evaluated for **Lisfranc sprain** or FX. Nondisplaced **avulsion** FX of fifth metatarsal tuberosity requires only supportive measures. FX of the proximal fifth metatarsal 1.5 cm distal to the base of the tuberosity (**Jones or Dancer** FX) needs aggressive management because of the risk of nonunion and avascular necrosis. Soft tissue infections range from **ingrown toenails** to a serious complication usually requiring hospitalization. Spontaneous pain, with swelling and erythema of first MTPJ, suggests gout

(cont.)

FOOT PAIN (cont.)

MANAGEMENT

- **Analgesia:** NSAIDs (see "Pain")
- RICE, buddy tape toe FX, rigid ortho shoe, posterior mold, crutches. Orthopedic consult for unstable or clinically significant FX. Ingrown toenail: warm soaks, NSAIDs, Abx, definitive toenail avulsion
- **Diabetic ulcer infection:** saline dressing, possible debridement, control hyperglycemia, consider **cellulitis** or x-ray to R/O **osteomyelitis.** Vancomycin 20 mg/kg IV BID plus ampicillin/sulbactam 3 g IV or piperacillin/tazobactam 4.5 g IV QID

DICTATION/DOCUMENTATION

- **General:** level of distress
- **VS and SaO$_2$** (if indicated)
- **Foot/Toes:** Pt is able to bear weight and ambulate with/without pain. There is no obvious asymmetry or deformity of the R/L foot when compared to the R/L foot. No surface trauma, ecchymosis, erythema, lesions, ulcers, or breaks in skin integrity. No bony step-off or deformity, no tenderness to palpation over toes, mid foot, or hind foot, or sole. Normal plantar/dorsiflexion, inversion/eversion. Distal motor and neurovascular status are intact

X-RAY NOTE

For example, right foot x-ray series was done to R/O FX or dislocation. There was no FX, dislocation, soft tissue swelling, or foreign body noted

SPLINT NOTE

There was no neurovascular compromise after splint/boot application; the splint/ boot was in good alignment and the pt had good sensation and cap refill at the time of discharge If unable to bear weight—crutches, then recheck 1 to 2 days

⊃TIP

- **Maltreatment:** location/pattern of injury, correlation of story to injury, degree/extent of injury. Suspect maltreatment with certain transverse, oblique, and/or spiral FXs; bilateral and/or symmetrical FXs; epiphyseal separations, bruising, or injuries in various stages of healing or injuries that are not consistent with the MOI. Lower extremity injuries that are highly specific for maltreatment include metaphyseal–epiphyseal FXs

DON'T MISS!

- Hair tourniquet in infants/children
- Lisfranc FXs
- Vascular occlusion

CHILD WITH LIMP

HX

▧ Bilateral versus unilateral
▧ Duration—acute versus chronic
▧ Trauma
▧ Fever/infection
▧ Pain characteristics—constant, intermittent, night pain, awaken from sleep
▧ Aggravating/relieving factors
▧ Associated symptoms—morning stiffness, incontinence, sciatica, leg weakness, back pain, recent use of antibiotics, recent illness (e.g., strep pharyngitis or viral illness)
▧ Risk factors for maltreatment/interpersonal/family violence (see "Maltreatment")

AGES 1 TO 3

▧ **Minor trauma:** most common such as contusion, sprain, wound or lesion on foot, or hair tourniquet. FXs less common; consider maltreatment. **Toddler FX** may occur in unsteady younger children learning to walk and run. This tibial FX can be spiral or oblique and is usually nondisplaced and the fibula is not involved. **Transient toxic synovitis:** inability to bear weight resulting from pain caused by transient inflammation of the synovium of the hip joint. Common cause of unilateral nontraumatic hip or groin pain; may be referred to thigh or knee. Well-appearing child with recent viral infection in most cases; may have low grade fever. Holds hip flexed with slight abduction and external rotation. Pain with gentle log rolling of leg is significant. Usually self-limiting and responds to analgesia. Consider septic arthritis or osteomyelitis. Full exam needed to identify viral causes, back pain (discitis), abd etiology (appendicitis), GU (hernia, torsion), or other injuries. For new-onset limp in well child, diagnostic tests are often deferred to watchful waiting and follow-up in 24 hours. Possible CBC, ESR, CRP, UA; bilateral hip x-rays with frog view. **Septic arthritis:** orthopedic emergency that can lead to permanent damage. Usually febrile, ill-appearing child with inability to bear weight. Monoarticular—hip or knee most common. Joint is tender, red, warm, with decreased and painful ROM; swelling of hip can be difficult to assess. Hip flexed, abducted, and externally rotated; knee held in flexion. Diagnostics include CBC, ESR (>40), CRP, blood culture, arthrocentesis, x-rays, or other imaging. **Osteomyelitis:** acute bone infection often spread by bacteria from the bloodstream. Often high fever, irritable, malaise, poor intake, decreased and painful ROM. Joint erythema, swelling, tenderness

AGES 4 TO 10

▧ **FXs:** more common—minor strain, contusion. **Transient toxic synovitis:** possible until about age 10 years
▧ **Legg–Calve–Perthes disease:** also called AVN of the femoral head—collapse of hip joint and deformity of the femoral head. More common in boys, 4:1. Achy pain in hip, groin, or back of knee; painful ROM of hip, especially internal rotation and abduction. X-rays show small, flattened, fragmented femoral head
▧ **Cancer:** leukemia, osteosarcoma. **Discitis:** inflammatory Dx of intervertebral disc space. Pain radiates to legs; other signs include limp and unable to bear weight. Spine very tender to palpation

(cont.)

CHILD WITH LIMP (cont.)

AGES 11 TO TEENS

▨ **Trauma:** commonly caused by sports, MCV, or assault. **Osgood–Schlatter disease:** benign, self-limiting pain and edema of tibial tubercle; outside knee joint; no effusion. More common in active boys during rapid growth. Usually unilateral; pain, swelling, or tenderness just below patella. Improves with rest; exacerbated with jumping, kneeling, squatting, or using stairs. **SCFE:** posterior slip of femoral head from its neck at weak growth plate; more common in boys, Blacks, and the obese. Sudden or gradual onset. Holds leg in external rotation and has pain with internal rotation. Pain in hip, medial thigh, or referred only to knee. External rotation when attempting to flex hip. AP/lateral/frog-leg x-rays; lateral femoral neck line (Klein's line) will not cross femoral head; wide, irregular physis. Also consider: **gonococcal arthritis, HSP, SCD, SLE, RA, malignancy, intra-abd or GU causes, abuse**

PE

▨ See "General Template"—depends on underlying cause
▨ **Extrems:** musculoskeletal—muscle strength, muscular atrophy, joint tenderness, bony tenderness, bony deformity, joint effusions, passive and active range of motion, hip rotation
▨ **Galeazzi test:** measure the length of the femur with pt on his or her back, legs in adduction with hips, and knees both flexed at 90°. Knees should be in the same location. Short limbs may be a sign of occult fracture, dislocation, or developmental dysplasia of the hip. Ellis test—evaluate the length of the tibia by holding knees and medial malleoli together and checking the position of the knee

MDM/DDx

Children with limp often have undetected minor trauma, such as **contusions, sprains,** toddler FX, or **infection,** such as **ingrown toenails. Accidental physeal FX** and **maltreatment** must be considered. The history of recent viral illness supports the common etiology of **viral synovitis.** More serious causes of pediatric limp are **osteomyelitis, septic arthritis, bacterial synovitis,** or **diskitis.** Less common are **AVN, malignancy, RA,** or **intra-abd causes.** Other differentials also include **anemia, sickle cell ankle injury, soft tissue injury, appendicitis, acute arthritis, rheumatoid back pain (mechanical), insect bites, brain abscess, cat scratch disease, erythema multiforme, ankle FXs, femur FXs, foot FXs, hip FXs, knee FXs, pelvic FXs, tibia/fibula FXs, juvenile gout, hemophilia (Type A or B), IBD, Legg–Calve–Perthes disease neoplasms, spinal cord disorder, meningitis,** and **encephalitis, SCD,** or **rheumatic fever**

MANAGEMENT

▨ **Analgesia** (see "Pain"), reexamine
▨ No evidence of trauma "sick" C/O pain: pain/fever control, x-rays; labs: CBC, ESR, CRP, blood Cxs
▨ Trauma: RICE, x-rays
▨ **Imaging:**
   ▨ X-rays: AP and lateral/frog-leg view of the pelvis
   ▨ Possible MRI
   ▨ Ultz (joint effusions), consider joint aspiration
   ▨ Consider septic joint, SCFE, or AVN
   ▨ Long leg posterior splint for toddler FX and x-ray again in 2 weeks for callus formation

(cont.)

CHILD WITH LIMP (cont.)

DICTATION/DOCUMENTATION

- **General:** level of distress
- **VS and SaO$_2$**
- **Extrem:** the pt is able to bear weight with/without pain. There is/is not obvious asymmetry or deformity of the R/L leg when compared to the R/L leg. No surface trauma, ecchymosis, erythema, lesions, or ulcers noted, including sole of foot. No bony step-off or deformity, and no tenderness to palpation of leg. Normal flexion/extension, abduction/adduction, or internal and external log roll of hip. Knee is NT, FROM, no STS or effusion, popliteal fossa NT without swelling. Ankle, foot, and toes are NT with normal FROM. Gait is antalgic/Trendelenburg/waddling/stiff-legged/toe walking/steppage/slow. Distal motor and neurovascular status is intact. Include abd, back, groin, and GU exam

X-RAY NOTE

There was no FX, dislocation, soft tissue swelling, or foreign body noted

SPLINT NOTE

There was no neurovascular compromise after splint application; the splint was in good alignment and the pt had good sensation and capillary refill at the time of discharge

▶ TIPS

- Suspect maltreatment with certain transverse, oblique, and/or spiral FXs; bilateral and/or symmetrical FXs; epiphyseal separations, bruising, or injuries in various stages of healing or injuries that are not consistent with the MOI
- Limp can be caused by pathology of the CNS, back, leg, abd, or GU system
- The location of pain does not always reflect the location of pathology

DON'T MISS!

- **Maltreatment:** location/pattern of injury, correlation of story as previously noted to injury, degree/extent of injury

SALTER HARRIS GROWTH PLATE FRACTURES

SALTR

I   S = Same/Straight
II A = Above
III L = Lower
IV T = Through
V   R = Rammed/Crushed

MEB

M   Metaphysis
E   Epiphysis
B   Both

Normal	Type I	Type II	Type III	Type IV	Type V
	Straight across	Above	Lower or BeLow	Two or Through	Erasure of Growth plate or Crush

R.Medina.12

Salter Harris growth plate fractures

LACERATIONS/WOUNDS

HX

- Exact time of injury/delayed presentation/prior treatment
- MOI: blunt, penetrating, crush injury, organic matter, animal bite, FB
- Dominant hand, occupation, work related
- Puncture wound through tennis shoe (*Pseudomonas*)
- Contaminated with sea water
- High-pressure paint gun, staple gun
- Closed-fist wounds
- Associated injury, self-inflicted wounds
- HX: comorbidities: DM, immunosuppressed
- Meds
- Allergies
- Tetanus immunization status
- Accidental/maltreatment trauma/interpersonal violence

PE

- **General:** level of distress, pain, F/C
- **VS and SaO$_2$**
- **Skin:** wound location, length, depth, linear, curvilinear, stellate, flap, jagged
    - Tissue loss, devitalized tissue, visible or palpable FB
    - Crush injury, exposed bone or tendon, active bleeding, STS, ecchymosis
- **Neuro:**
    - Distal motor neurovascular status
    - Repeat motor exam under anesthesia and ROM

MDM/DDx

Wounds are divided into types of repair: **simple, intermediate**, or **complex.** Anatomic location and wound length in cm must also be noted. Multiple wounds can be reported in total cm unless the wounds are of varying complexity. **Simple repair** includes closure of superficial wounds involving only the skin, regardless of length. Intermediate lacerations include approximation of skin and subcutaneous layer, galia, or superficial fascia. Simple wound closure that requires extensive cleaning and removal of particulate matter may be classified as intermediate in some cases. **Complex repair** includes multiple layer repair, debridement, extensive undermining, or placement of retention sutures

(cont.)

LACERATIONS/WOUNDS (cont.)

MANAGEMENT

- ▦ Thorough wound irrigation and exploration with adequate hemostasis is the foundation of wound care. Identification of underlying deep-structure injury or retained FB is essential for optimal wound healing
  - ▦ X-ray for possible FB
  - ▦ Update tetanus status
  - ▦ Consider Abx for contaminated wounds; delayed presentation or immunosuppressed pts may require anxiolytic agent for wound repair (PO or intranasal)
- ▦ Refer/Consult for pts with:
  - ▦ Large avulsions or near amputations
  - ▦ Severe crush injuries and/or devitalized tissue
  - ▦ Involvement of eyelid tarsal plate or tear duct system
  - ▦ Auricular hematoma
  - ▦ Large cartilage defects

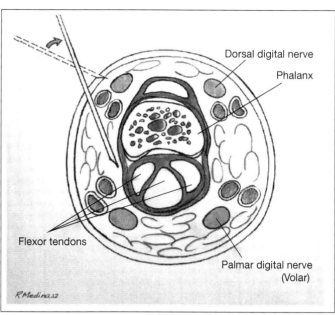

Cross-section depicting digital nerve block anatomy

(cont.)

LACERATIONS/WOUNDS (cont.)

SUTURE REMOVAL

- ◼ 4 to 5 days: eyelid, lip, face
- ◼ 4 to 6 days: pinna ear, neck
- ◼ 7 days: scalp/head
- ◼ 7 to 10 days: trunk or extremity
- ◼ 12 to 14 days: hand or foot

LACERATION PROCEDURE NOTE:

Procedure explained and consent obtained. The wound was anesthetized with _____mL of _____ with good anesthesia. (Note local topical anesthesia, local infiltration, field block, digital block, metacarpal head block.) Sterile drape and prep were done. Copious irrigation was done with NS and the wound explored. (Note whether able to visualize depth of wound.) There was no foreign body or deep-structure injury noted. (Note whether examined under range of motion.) Wound edges were approximated with good alignment using _____ (sutures, staples, skin adhesive, skin tapes).

There were (number) of sutures/staples placed with (type of) suture. Note type of dressing applied if done. Tolerated procedure well with no complications

⊙ TIPS

- ◼ A detailed motor neurovascular/tendon exam if injury to digit/extremity
- ◼ Advise pt/parent of retained FB and document
- ◼ If wound is healing poorly or infected consider retained FB

DON'T MISS!

- ◼ Open FX, tendon/nerve injuries, joint capsule disruption, neurovascular disruption
- ◼ **Maltreatment:** location/pattern of injury, correlation of the story to the injury, and degree or extent of injury

CUTANEOUS ABSCESS/CELLULITIS

HX

- Age of the pt
- Onset, duration
- Progression since onset of symptoms
- Precipitating factors (injury, insect bite)
- Systemic symptoms (fever, feeding, hydration, irritability)
- Past medical history (previous abscess, immunocompromised)
- Contacts with similar symptoms (MRSA risk factors, overcrowding, poverty)
- Comorbidities, especially immunosuppression
- Immunization status

PE

- **General:** WDWN, alert, hydration, ill appearing
- **VS and SaO$_2$**
- **Skin:** local signs of acute infection, erythema, swelling, warmth, tenderness, induration, fluctuance, regional lymphadenopathy

MDM/DDx

MRSA is the leading cause of skin and soft tissue infections and occurs frequently in children. Children under the age of 2 are at increased risk of MRSA infection. Other children at risk include those with eczema, frequent insect bites, obesity, and prior history of MRSA infections. I&D is the definitive treatment required for both diagnosis and treatment of an abscess. I&D is often the only treatment necessary in an abscess <5 cm in diameter in a well child with minimal systemic symptoms. Very large **abscesses** or those with **cellulitis** require antibiotic therapy; possible admission for IV Abx. More serious abscess locations are over a joint or near the orbit and may require IV Abx for full penetration.

MANAGEMENT: ABSCESS

- If pt is toxic appearing: CBC with diff, chem panel, blood CRP
- Bedside ultz to distinguish between cellulitis and abscess
- I&D— adequate I&D is foundation of treatment; usually no packing needed or possible wick only to keep wound open; wound C&S (controversial)
- Warm soaks
- NSAIDs
- Oral analgesia or procedural sedation in addition to local anesthesia; oral or intranasal anxiolytic or conscious sedation may be required for large abscesses

Abscess Severity

- *Mild*—I&D only (Abx not usually indicated unless the pt is also immunosuppressed [e.g., DM, CA, Hep C, HIV], MRSA, multiple abscesses, cellulitis)
- *Moderate*—Abx (7–10 days): Bactrim DS PO BID or doxycycline 100 mg PO BID; if clindamycin 450 mg TID is used for PCN allergy, watch for GI SXS
- *Severe*—Vancomycin 15 to 20 mg/kg IV QID
- Consult for perirectal abscess
- Tetanus: adults >19 years, substitute 1-time dose of Tdap for Td booster; then boost with Td every 10 years

(cont.)

CUTANEOUS ABSCESS/CELLULITIS (cont.)

MANAGEMENT: CELLULITIS

- Consider hyperglycemia
- Fever control, NSAIDs, analgesia, elevation, and warm soaks
- Possible soft tissue x-ray or ultz to R/O FB or gas
- Abx (7–10 days)

Abscess Severity

Mild—amoxicillin/clavulanate 875 mg PO BID, cephalexin 500 mg PO QID. If clindamycin 450 mg TID is used for PCN allergy, watch for GI SXS

Moderate/Severe—IV PCN, Rocephin, clindamycin (severe pts—admit)

- Tetanus: adults >19 years, substitute 1-time dose of Tdap for Td booster; then boost with Td every 10 years
- **Erysipelas:** cephalexin 500 mg PO QID X 10 days or clindamycin 600 mg QID X 5 days then decrease to 300 mg QID; 10-day course for other
- Recheck 1 to 2 days, sooner if worse
- Address underlying condition that may predispose to cellulitis such as chronic venous insufficiency or lymphedema
- Admit for IV Abx if immunosuppressed, extensive, rapid spread, failed outpatient, toxic

SUPERFICIAL CUTANEOUS ABSCESS I&D PROCEDURE NOTE

Procedure explained, and consent obtained. The wound was anesthetized with _____ mL of _____ with good anesthesia. Sterile drape and prep were done. The fluctuant center was incised with #11 blade scalpel. A small/moderate/large amount of (exudate/blood/caseous material) was expressed or removed. The wound was probed for loculated areas and irrigated with normal saline. Note whether the wound was packed loosely with wick or left open. DSD was applied. Tolerated procedure well with no complications

▶ TIP

- Possible admission of even well-appearing child if large abscess (>5 cm) or serious location

DON'T MISS!

- Necrotizing fasciitis especially in immunocompromised pts

PAIN

The appropriate management of acute pediatric pain is a priority in the urgent and emergency setting. Although most instances of pain are caused by **acute injury** or **illness**, some children present with **chronic diseases** that cause pain such as cancer, rheumatoid arthritis, and sickle cell anemia. In addition, iatrogenic causes of pain, such as venipuncture and injections, should be considered. Children may experience heightened reactions to pain because of anxiety and fear or inability to communicate. Unfortunately, children in pain may be at risk for **inadequate pain management** for a variety of reasons. Infants and preverbal children can be challenging to assess and may not be able to localize, understand, or communicate their complaint of pain. Misconceptions persist about the use of opioids in children and concern about side effects, respiratory depression, and addiction. **The goal of pediatric pain management is not only immediate relief but to minimize the potential future negative impact related to the pain experience**. Oral, intranasal, or IV administration is recommended to avoid the trauma of "a shot" to a child already in pain

ASSESSMENT

Accurate age-related assessment of pain is performed using standardized scoring tools that include objective findings in the infant or preverbal child and self-report scales for older children. Pain should be assessed at the same time as VS.

- **Newborns:** Premature Infant Pain Profile assessment parameters include indicators of infant pain similar to the Crying Requires oxygen Increased VS Expression Sleep (CRIES) Scale, that is, high-pitched cry, SaO_2 <95%, VS (elevated heart rate or B/P), facial expression (brow bulge, grimace, squeezing eyes shut, deepened nasolabial fold), opening lips/mouth, sleeplessness; or use CRIES Postoperative Pain Scale
- **>2 Month:** Face, Legs, Activity, Cry, Consolability (FLACC) Scale
- **>3 Years:** Poker Chip Scale, Wong–Baker FACES Scale, FACES Pain Scale—Revised (FPS-R)
- **Children 8 to 11 years:** use visual analog tools on a horizontal or numeric scale Children may be assessed using the revised FACES Pain Scale or the 10-cm Visual Analog Scale
- **Adolescents:** use numerical self-report (0–10) rating scale without an accessory pain assessment tool

MANAGEMENT

- Physical, behavioral, or cognitive measures include psychological and emotional support, caregiver presence and education, distraction techniques or rewards, and age-appropriate coping strategies
- 12% to 25% sucrose solution (with or without a pacifier) to decrease neonatal distress during painful procedures (e.g., venipuncture)

LOCAL PAIN MANAGEMENT

- Vibrating devices (e.g., Buzzy pain relief system)
- Cold packs (also see "Wound and Lacerations")

(cont.)

PAIN (cont.)

MEDICATIONS

- **Acetaminophen:** well tolerated, often adequate for mild to moderate pain
  - 10 to 15 mg/kg every 4 hours PRN; less frequent in neonates
  - Limit daily intake to avoid hepatotoxicity: premature 45 mg/kg/d; neonate <10 days 60 mg/kg/d; children 75 mg/kg/d. Daily cumulative dose should not exceed 100 mg/kg/d in children and 75 mg/kg/d in infants
  - Rectal: slower and variable onset of action; increase dosage to 20 mg/kg and may use loading dose of up to 40 mg/kg
  - Intravenous administration approved in children. Intravenous: 2 to 12 years of age—single dose 15 mg/kg every 6 hours, then 12.5 mg/kg every 4 hours, to a max of 75 mg/kg/d
- **NSAIDs:** well tolerated and appropriate for mild to moderate pain >6 months of age. Ibuprofen is the preferred NSAID in children because it is equally effective as others with fewer side effects.
  - 10 mg/kg every 6 to 8 hours to a maximum of 40 mg/kg/d
  - Toradol 0.5 mg/kg to a maximum of 15 mg or 1 mg/kg IM to a max of 30 mg
- **Aspirin:** avoid in infants and children due to risk of Reye's syndrome
- **Opioids:** safe in most children; use with caution in children <6 months due to delayed elimination and immature central respiratory control. Monitor for respiratory depression or apnea with even small opioid doses
- **Codeine:** poorly tolerated due to GI upset and constipation. Can be combined with acetaminophen in children over 3 years
  - Oral solution contains 12 mg codeine/120 mg acetaminophen per 5 mL
  - 3 to 6 years 5 mL q4 to 6h; 7 to 12 years 10 mL q4 to 6h; 12+ years 15 mL q4 to 6h
- **Lortab elixir:** decreased amount of acetaminophen and volume; often better tolerated than acetaminophen and codeine
  - 2 to 3 years old (12 to 15 kg) 2.8 mL q4 to 6h; 4 to 6 years old (16–22 kg) 3.75 mL q4 to 6h; 7 to 9 years old (23–31 kg) 5.6 mL q4 to 6h; 10 to 13 years old (32–45 kg) 7.5 mL q4 to 6h; 14 + (46 kg and up) 11.25 mL q4 to 6h
- **Morphine:** safe choice in children, rapid onset, short duration of 2 to 4 hours. May also be used as a continuous infusion or pt-controlled infusion in an older pt.
  - Neonates 0.05 to 0.2 mg/kg q4h; infants and children 0.1 to 0.2 mg /kg IV q2 to 4h; adolescent 2.5 to 5.0 mg q2 to 4h
- **Meperidine:** avoid due to possible seizures and toxic metabolites
- **Intranasal fentanyl:** rapid onset, effective. 1.5 mcg/kg (100 mcg max dose)
- **Intranasal versed:** 0.2 to 0.5 mg/kg (10 mg max dose)
- **Local or topical anesthetics:** helpful in minimizing pain caused by procedures such as venipuncture or IV insertion, lumbar puncture
  - EMLA (lidocaine and prilocaine cream): use may be limited due to slow onset of action (30–90 min)
  - Numby Stuff™: electrical field used to distribute lidocaine into small area of deep tissue (iontophoresis); onset about 15 min
  - Local infiltration with 1% lidocaine prior to venous or arterial cannulation; less pain experienced when buffered with sodium bicarbonate (4 mL lidocaine: 1 mL sodium bicarbonate)

(cont.)

PAIN (cont.)

◎ TIPS

- In addition to pain management, procedural sedation may also be indicated (e.g., complex lacerations, orthopedic, and other minor procedures). Sedation/hypnotics may be used along with short-acting medications (e.g., propofol with ketamine)
- Skin-to-skin contact/family presence can be helpful in the ED setting

DON'T MISS!

- Respiratory depression/hypotension with opioid use naloxone (Narcan) as reversal agent

FEVER

The approach to pediatric fever depends on the age of the child, level of toxicity, immunization status, and clinical findings. An elevated temperature of 38°C is considered fever in pediatric patients

HX

- Prematurity, low birth weight, prolonged rupture of membranes, fetal hypoxia, limp, seizure at birth
- Maternal HX: pregnancy HX, delivery details, postpartum fever, illnesses, STI, HIV, Hep C, neonatal death of previous child because of infection, hospitalization, surgery, Abx use
- Poor feeding, fussy, irritable, lethargic, apparent pain, sleeping changes
- F/C, N/V
- Rash, lesions, jaundice, pallor
- Urinary output, wet diapers, stools
- Runny nose, cough, earache, sore throat
- Circumcised male infant, toilet trained, bed wetting
- Sick contacts, day care, close contact vaccination status, homelessness or inability to care for infant, travel or exposure to others with recent travel

PE

- **General:** WDWN, awake and active. Interacts appropriately with surroundings and examiner, in no acute distress or toxic appearing. Normal, weak, or shrill cry. Growth parameters with percentiles. Note weight in kg and birth weight
- **VS and SaO$_2$:** fever 38°C, tachycardia, tachypnea
- **Skin:** PWD, texture and turgor, cap refill. Pallor, jaundice, cyanosis, mottling. Rash, lesions, mucocutaneous vesicles, petechiae
- **HEENT:**
  - **Head:** normocephalic. Fontanels (if still open)
  - **Eyes:** moist and bright. Sclera and conjunctivae normal. PERRLA, EOMI, or tracks normally
  - **Ears:** pre- or postauricular lymphadenopathy or erythema. Canals clear or erythema, edema, exudate. TMs normal or erythematous, bulging, retraction, fluid level, bullae, perforation
  - **Nose:** patent, rhinorrhea, erythema, nasal flaring
  - **Mouth/Throat:** MMM, posterior pharynx clear or erythema, exudate, lesions
- **Neck:** supple, FROM, meningismus, lymphadenopathy
- **Chest:** respiratory unlabored, adequate tidal volume or tachypnea, retractions, accessory muscle use, grunting, stridor, head bobbing. CTA; wheezes, crackles, or rhonchi. SaO$_2$ ___% >95% on room air. Dry or congested cough noted
- **Heart:** RRR, no murmurs, rubs, or gallops
- **Abd:** soft, nondistended. BSA+. Tenderness, rebound, rigidity, masses, organomegaly. Active vomiting
- **Back:** no spinal or CVAT
- **GU:** normal external genitalia—note whether circumcised. Wet diaper. Rash or lesions. Femoral pulses, inguinal lymphadenopathy, hernia
- **Extremities:** symmetric, no deformity. Moves all extrems with good strength, FROM. Neurovascularly intact. No cyanosis, edema, mottling. No obvious joint irritability. Able to bear weight if appropriate
- **Neuro:** alert, active, and developmentally normal for age. GCS 15. Muscle tone good and equal, bilaterally. No focal neuro deficits

(cont.)

FEVER (cont.)

MDM/DDx

SBI in pediatric pts requires a high index of suspicion, thorough history, and meticulous physical exam. In the very young, signs of systemic infection are often vague and nonspecific. Febrile neonates (<28 days) are at significant risk for SBI and must have a complete septic workup and be admitted even if well appearing. Neonates who present with signs of toxicity have up to 20% risk for SBI. Well-appearing but febrile infants (28–90 days) may sometimes be discharged home with very close F/U if the workup is negative for SBI and empiric parenteral Abx given. Diagnostics for children 3 months to 3 years with fever is based on stability or toxicity and immunization status. Lower risk is associated with WBC 5K to 15K and <20% bands (but is not a reliable single test) and a negative UA. Incomplete vaccinations for *Streptococcus pneumoniae* or **H-flu type B should be noted as risk factors for SBI**. Concern for **UTI** is high for all febrile female infants and toddlers and males < 6 months or uncircumcised males <12 months. UTI is often associated with **bacteremia** in children <60 days. Febrile infants with UTI often also have signs of failure to thrive, irritability or lethargy, and possible jaundice. Urine obtained by catheterization is required to avoid contamination. **Pyelonephritis** may be present in up to 20% of infants with urine negative for pyuria, and urine culture is needed. **Neonatal sepsis** occurring in the first days of life can result in septic shock. Sepsis after the first week is often caused by bacterial **meningitis**. The incidence of bacterial meningitis is highest in the first 30 days of life. Meningismus or nuchal rigidity is difficult to detect in neonates and infants and classic signs of meningitis may be minimal or absent, but a bulging fontanel is common. Other causes of neonatal SBI include **sinusitis, pneumonia, omphalitis, soft tissue infection, joint** or **bone infection, E. coli infection, HSV, and strep B sepsis**. Young children with rapid elevation of fever are at risk for **febrile seizures**. Acute **viral illness** is common at every age and ranges from benign coryza to severe **bronchiolitis**. Care must be taken to exclude SBI requiring Abx and admission, **dehydration**, or **impending respiratory failure**

(cont.)

FEVER (cont.)

MANAGEMENT

- Fever control
  - **Acetaminophen:** <12 years: 10 to 15 mg/kg PO q6 to 8h PRN, not to exceed 2.6 g/d (5 doses/24 hr); >12 years: 40 to 60 mg/kg/d PO divided q6h PRN, not to exceed 3.75 g/d (5 doses/24 hr). Avoid higher doses that can lead to impaired renal function
  - **Ibuprofen:** 6 months to 12 years: <102.5°F: 5 to 10 mg/kg/dose PO q6 to 8h, not to exceed 40 mg/kg/d; >102.5°F: 10 mg/kg/dose q6 to 8h, not to exceed 40 mg/kg/d
- Neonates (<28 days)
  - Complete septic workup required in all cases of fever in neonates <28 days
  - CBC with diff, chem panel, cath UA, blood and urine culture, stool culture (if blood, mucus, diarrhea), LP; CXR in most cases; do if tachycardia, low SaO₂, cough, SOB; RSV nasal washing if indicated
  - Meds: ampicillin 50 mg/kg *plus* cefotaxime 50 mg/kg or gentamicin 2.5 mg/kg
  - Add acyclovir if maternal HX HSV, seizures, mucocutaneous vesicles, increased cell count (especially WBC) on CSF
  - Admit
- Infants (28–60 days) with fever >38°C (100.4°F)
  - **Toxic:** same workup as neonate and **admit**
  - **Nontoxic:** essentially same workup as neonate—include LP if WBC or UA not normal
  - Can discharge if well appearing, WBC 5K to 15K and <20% bands, negative UA, close F/U, good instructions
- Infants (2–6 months) with fever >38°C (100.4°F)
  - **Toxic:** same workup as neonate and **admit**. Ceftriaxone *or* cefotaxime 50 to 100 mg/kg; vancomycin 15 mg/kg if concern for bacterial meningitis
  - **Nontoxic + immunized:** UA/Cx, CXR. Discharge with Abx if indicated and close F/U
  - **Nontoxic, *not* immunized:** UA/Cx, CBC with diff, CXR. Ceftriaxone 50 mg/kg if WBC >15K
  - Add LP and blood cultures in most cases. Discharge with close F/U
- Infants 6 months–child 3 years with fever >38°C (100.4°F). Some experts have threshold of 39°C (102.2°F)
  - **Toxic:** same workup as neonate and **admit**. Ceftriaxone *or* cefotaxime 50 to 100 mg/kg; vancomycin 15 mg/kg if concern for bacterial meningitis
  - **Nontoxic + immunized:** UA/UCx, CXR. Discharge with Abx if indicated and close F/U
  - **Nontoxic, *not* immunized:** UA/UCx, CBC with diff, CXR. Ceftriaxone 50 mg/kg if WBC > 15K
  - Add LP and blood cultures in most cases. Discharge with close F/U
  - **If the child is well appearing with fever >38°C to 39°C (100.4°F to 102.2°F):** possible UA and CXR, discharge with specific instructions to return for worsening SXS and close F/U

(cont.)

FEVER (cont.)

DICTATION/DOCUMENTATION

- **General:** WDWN child, awake and active. Not toxic appearing. Interacts appropriately with surroundings and examiner, in no acute distress
- **VS and SaO$_2$:** febrile, tachycardia, tachypnea, hypoxia
- **Skin:** PWD, normal texture and turgor without rash or cyanosis. No scaling, blistering, peeling, desquamation. No petechiae or purpura
- **HEENT:**
  - **Head:** normocephalic, AT. Fontanels normal (if still open)
  - **Eyes:** moist and bright. Sclera and conjunctivae normal; no injection, tearing, or discharge. PERRLA, EOMI. No nystagmus or diplopia noted
  - **Ears:** canals clear without erythema, edema, exudate. Patent. TMs clear; no erythema, bulging, retraction. No pre- or postauricular lymphadenopathy or erythema
  - **Nose:** patent without rhinorrhea or nasal flaring
  - **Mouth/Throat:** lips moist, MMM, no strawberry tongue, posterior pharynx clear without lesions, erythema, or exudate. Strong suck or able to swallow fluids
- **Neck:** supple, FROM, no meningismus or lymphadenopathy
- **Chest:** respirations easy and unlabored, normal TV. No retractions or accessory muscle use noted. No grunting, head bobbing, or stridor. Lungs clear to auscultation; no wheezes, crackles, or rhonchi. SaO$_2$ ____%, which is within normal limits (if 95% or >)
- **Heart:** RRR, tones normal, no murmurs, rubs, or gallops
- **Abd:** round, nondistended. BSA. No tenderness, rebound, rigidity to palpation. No masses or organomegaly palpated
- **Back:** no spinal or CVAT
- **GU:** normal external genitalia without rash. No inguinal lymphadenopathy or hernia noted
- **Extremities:** FROM, good strength bilaterally. Neurovascular intact. No cyanosis or edema
- **Neuro:** alert, active, and developmentally normal for age. GCS 15. Muscle tone good and equal, bilaterally. No focal neurological findings noted

O TIPS

- Higher concern for neonates and infants if preterm, postnatal illness/hospitalization, systemic disease, Abx therapy. Diligent search for focal source of infection and child appears well hydrated
- WBC 5,000 to 15,000 with <1,500 bands, normal UA, and urine Gram stain is reassuring (normal CXR; stool smear)
- Must have reliable caregiver and close F/U

DON'T MISS!

- Females and uncircumcised males ages 6 to 24 months: obtain UA/Cx; circumcised males: obtain UA/Cx until 12 months
- Discharge if stable and treat UTI or other focal infection as needed

MALTREATMENT

HX

Begin the history with open-ended questions about how the injury occurred, and proceed to more specific questions. Begin the history with the child and the caregiver together, and then separate them. Repeated questioning can be perceived by young children as implying their initial answer was incorrect and may lead to a changing history. Avoid yes/no questions; document questions and answers using direct quotes.

- Time of injury, MOI (elevation and motion, mechanics of the injurious circumstances)
- Is history consistent with injury (specific and detailed)?
- Is history consistent with development age of the child?
- Are there any unexplained injuries?
- Behavior before, during, and after the injury
- Alteration in LOC
- Caregiver with child at the time of injury
- PMH: trauma, hospitalizations, congenital conditions, chronic illnesses
- FH: bleeding, metabolic, genetic, bone, or mental health disorders
- Pregnancy HX: planned/unplanned, prenatal care, postnatal complications, postpartum depression
- Familial pattern of discipline
- PH of child maltreatment to pt, siblings, parents
- Substance abuse by caregivers in the home
- SH: financial stressors and resources
- Risk factors for maltreatment/interpersonal/family violence

(cont.)

MALTREATMENT (cont.)

PE

- **General:** appearance, hygiene, mental status
- **VS and SaO$_2$:** tachycardia or bradycardia (significant for shock/neurogenic shock), widening pulse pressure
- **Skin:** PWD, cool, moist, pale; location, size, shape of bruises, burns, bites, patterned injuries, injuries in various stages of healing
- **HEENT:**
  - **Head:** surface trauma, alopecia, bulging anterior fontanel TTP, bony step-off
  - **Eyes:** PERRLA, EOMI, periorbital ecchymosis
  - **Ears:** canals patent. TMs, Battle's sign, hemotympanum. CSF leak
  - **Nose:** nasal injury, septal hematoma, epistaxis, CSF rhinorrhea
  - **Face:** facial trauma
  - **Mouth/Throat:** intraoral trauma, bruising, petechiae, frenulum tear, teeth and mandible stable
- **Neck:** FROM without limitation or pain, NT to firm palp at midline
- **Chest:** NT, CTA
- **Heart:** RRR, no murmur, gallop, rub, clear tones
- **Abd:** surface trauma, BSA, NT
- **Back:** no spinal or CVAT
- **Pelvis:** NT to palpation and stable to compression, femoral pulses strong and equal
- **GU: see "Genitourinary Pain"**
- **Female:** SMR, inspection of the labia majora, labia minora, introitus, and hymen for erythema, lesions, abrasions, or tears. Include hymen for configuration, lacerations, transections, absence of tissue, bruising
  - Speculum exam for prepubescent females only if there is active bleeding; pubertal females with evidence of penetration
- **Male:** Inspect scrotum and penis for erythema, bruises, bite marks, abrasions, suction petechiae
  - Inspect urethral meatus for erythema, lacerations, and discharge
  - Perianal: Inspect for anal laxity, edema, bruises, lacerations, abrasions, discharge
- **Extremities:** FROM, NT, distal CMS intact
- **Neuro:** A&O ×3, GCS 15, no focal neuro deficits

MDM/DDx

A high index of suspicion for child maltreatment must be maintained. Medical providers are mandated reporters, and therefore legally responsible for reporting "suspicions" of child maltreatment. Consult with members of the multidisciplinary team (e.g., social work, department of social services, law enforcement, sexual assault nurse examiner). It is important to remember that findings that appear to indicate maltreatment may be the result of other causes. (See **Differential Diagnosis of Child Maltreatment Physical Abuse**.) Common mimickers. A detailed history must be obtained. Children less than 2 years of age are more difficult to assess, may be asymptomatic despite having a TBI, and are at risk of abusive head trauma

(cont.)

MALTREATMENT (cont.)

MANAGEMENT

- Address life-threatening injuries as first priority (ABCs)
- Approach to diagnostic workup is dictated by the HX and PE
- **Labs:** CBC with diff, chem panel, calcium and phosphate, LFTs, amylase/lipase, coags, UA, urine NAAT GC/chlamydia, Utox, UCG. Rectal, throat, urethral, or vaginal cultures for GC; rectal or vaginal cultures for chlamydia
- **X-rays:** skeletal survey <2 years with suspected physical abuse. For children >2 years, order specific x-rays as indicated. Unenhanced brain CT for all infants suspected of physical abuse and all children with evidence of head injury. Abd CT with IV contrast for children with evidence of intra-abd trauma or elevated LFTs, amylase, or lipase
- **Ophthalmologic exam:** complete dilated fundoscopic examination in all children <5 years if abusive head trauma suspected
- **Forensic evidence collection:** for alleged sexual abuse within the previous 72 hours; however, the yield is low and the majority of evidence is found on clothing and linens. When available, a specially trained health care provider should obtain this evidence

DICTATION/DOCUMENTATION

Documentation of each step of the evaluation and management of suspected child maltreatment is of critical importance. The medical record should be factual, stating direct quotes when possible. Describe injuries in as much detail as possible, using photographs when possible.

- **General:** level of distress, awake and alert; no odor of ETOH
- **VS and SaO$_2$**
- **Skin:** PWD, no surface trauma
- **HEENT:**
    - **Head:** atraumatic, no palpable deformities. Fontanel flat (if still open)
    - **Eyes:** PERRLA, EOMI, no periorbital ecchymosis. Fundoscopic exam
    - **Ears:** TMs clear, no hemotympanum or Battle's sign
    - **Nose/Face:** atraumatic, no epistaxis or septal hematoma. Facial bones symmetric, NT to palpation and stable with attempts at manipulation
    - **Mouth/Throat:** no intraoral trauma. Teeth and mandible are intact
- **Neck:** no point tenderness, step-off, or deformity to firm palpation of the cervical spine at the midline. No spasm or paraspinal muscle tenderness. No masses. FROM without limitation or pain
- **Chest:** no surface trauma or asymmetry. NT without crepitus or deformity. Normal tidal volume. Breath sounds clear bilaterally
- **Heart:** RRR, no murmurs, rubs, or gallops. All peripheral pulses are intact and equal
- **Abd:** nondistended without abrasions or ecchymosis. BSA+. No tenderness, guarding, or rebound. No masses. Good femoral pulses
- **Back:** no contusions, ecchymosis, or abrasions are noted. NT without step-off or deformity to firm palpation of the thoracic and lumbar spine
- **Pelvis:** NT to palpation and stable to compression
- **GU:** normal external genitalia with no blood at the meatus (if applicable)
- **Rectal:** normal tone. No rectal wall tenderness or mass. Stool is brown and heme negative (if applicable)
- **Extremities:** no surface trauma. FROM. Distal motor, neurovascular supply is intact
- **Neuro:** alert and oriented, GCS 15, CN II–XII grossly intact. Motor and sensory exam nonfocal. Reflexes are symmetric. Speech is clear and gait is steady

(cont.)

MALTREATMENT (cont.)

⊙ TIPS

- Suspect maltreatment with certain transverse, oblique, and/or spiral FXs; bilateral and/or symmetrical FXs; epiphyseal separations, bruising, burns, or injuries in various stages of healing or injuries that are not consistent with the MOI. Injuries that are highly specific for maltreatment include metaphyseal–epiphyseal FXs or pelvic FXs
- Obtain a skeletal survey and ophthalmology consult in siblings less than 2 years of age

DON'T MISS!

The Four Distinct Characteristics of Maltreatment	High-Risk Injuries for Child Maltreatment
<ul><li>Location of the injury</li><li>Pattern of the injury</li><li>Correlation of the story to the injury</li><li>Degree or extent of the injury</li></ul>	<ul><li>Bruises in children who cannot "cruise"</li><li>Bruises of the trunk, face, ear, neck, hand, feet, posterior legs, and buttocks</li><li>Long-bone FXs in children who do not walk</li><li>Rib FXs in children <1 year of age</li><li>Hollow viscus injury in children <4 years of age</li><li>Subdural hematomas in infants</li></ul>

DIFFERENTIAL DIAGNOSIS OF CHILD MALTREATMENT PHYSICAL ABUSE

Accidental Injury/Burns In Cultural Practices

- Cao gio (coining)
- Cupping
- Moxibustion
- Quat sha (spoon rubbing)

DERMATOLOGIC DISORDERS

- Mongolian spots
- Erythema multiforme
- Stevens–Johnson syndrome
- Fixed drug eruption
- Diaper dermatitis
- Phytophotodermatitis

GENETIC DISEASES

- Ehlers–Danlos syndrome
- Familial dysautonomia
- Vasculitis

(cont.)

MALTREATMENT (cont.)

GENITOURINARY DISORDERS

- Anal fissure
- Enlargement of hymenal opening
- Failure of midline fusion
- Lichen sclerosus
- *Molluscum contagiosum*
- Mongolian spots
- Nevi
- Perianal streptococcal dermatitis
- Straddle injury
- Urethral prolapse
- UTI
- Vaginal foreign body

HEMATOLOGIC DISORDERS

- ITP
- Leukemia
- Hemophilia
- Henoch–Schonlein purpura
- Vitamin K deficiency
- DIC

INFECTION

- Impetigo
- Staphylococcal scalded skin syndrome
- Sepsis
- Purpura fulminans (meningococcemia)

METABOLIC BONE DISEASE

- Osteogenesis imperfecta
- Copper deficiency
- Rickets

SYNCOPE

HX

- **Activities preceding/precipitating syncope:** postural changes (prolonged standing, change in position), hot showers, pain, or emotional stress may indicate vasovagal etiology (most common); physical exertion may indicate cardiac etiology; acute arousal or loud noises may indicate prolonged QT syndrome
- **Complete description of event:** prodrome of diaphoresis, light-headedness, nausea, dizziness, or visual changes common with vasovagal response; preceded by prolonged standing or change in position (sitting to standing), common with orthostasis; shortness of breath, chest pain, or palpitations common with cardiac etiology
- **Abnormal motor activity:** motor activity at the beginning of syncope, followed by prolonged time to return to baseline may indicate a seizure. Motor activity at the end of syncope common with vasovagal etiology
- **Past medical history:** congenital or acquired heart disease (e.g., Kawasaki syndrome, rheumatic heart disease), arrhythmia, previous syncope, diabetes, hypoglycemia, substance abuse, last normal menstrual period, sexual history
- **Family history:** cardiac disease, premature cardiac death (<50 years old), unexplained premature death in first- or second-degree relatives

PE

- **General:** age-related weight and size, level of activity and interaction
- **VS and SaO$_2$:** orthostatic intolerance, altered LOC, dry mucous membranes, cardiac murmur
- **Skin:** PWD, pallor, cyanosis, hydration
- **HEENT:**
  - **Head:** normocephalic without evidence of trauma. Fontanel normal (if still open)
  - **Eyes:** moist and bright. Sclera and conjunctivae normal. Pupils are equal, round, and reactive to light. Extraocular movements intact. No nystagmus or diplopia noted
  - **Ears:** canals patent. Tympanic membranes clear. No pre- or postauricular lymphadenopathy
  - **Nose:** patent without rhinorrhea or nasal flaring
  - **Mouth/Throat:** mucous membranes moist. Posterior pharynx clear without lesions, erythema, or exudates
- **Chest:** work of breathing, clear breath sounds without crackles, wheezes, or rhonchi
- **Heart:** RRR; presence of gallops, rubs, or murmurs
- **Abd:** soft, BSA, NT, without HSM
- **Extremities:** FROM with good strength, distal neurovascularly intact
- **Neuro:** awake, alert, GCS 15, age-appropriate behavior

MDM/DDx

In contrast to adults, **most causes of syncope** in the pediatric population are **benign. Vasovagal syncope** is the *most common cause* of syncope in children. However, syncope can be the result of more serious disease (**e.g., cardiac**) with the potential for sudden death. The goal in the ED is to identify life-threatening conditions, as well as those with the risk of significant injury. **Red flags for life-threatening causes of syncope** include: **family history of sudden cardiac death, syncope during exercise or while supine, associated chest pain or palpitations, abnormal EKG, abnormal cardiac examination, recurrent syncope, fall directly onto face, CHD, drugs with cardiac effect.** Diagnostic considerations include **hypoglycemia, seizure, pseudoseizure, complex migraine, breath-holding spells, self-strangulation or autoerotic asphyxia, malingering**

(cont.)

SYNCOPE (cont.)

MANAGEMENT

- Maintain ABCs
- Fasting blood sugar
- Hgb/Hct
- UCG for all postmenarcheal females, Utox if AMS
- EKG on all children with syncope, despite low diagnostic yield. Clinically significant findings: nonsinus rhythms, long or short corrected QT interval (QTc), delta wave, ventricular hypertrophy with strain, evidence of myocardial injury, Brugada syndrome (RSR in V1 and V2 with ST elevation)
- Brain CT scan if focal neurologic deficits, persistent AMS, or significant head injury as the result of syncope
- Echocardiogram, ambulatory EKG monitoring, exercise EKG, tilt-table test in consultation with a pediatric cardiologist

DICTATION/DOCUMENTATION

- **General:** WDWN child who is awake and active. Interacts appropriately with surroundings and examiner, in no acute distress
- **VS and SaO_2:** note VS and interpret as normal or abnormal, SaO_2 interpretation, weight in kg
- **Skin:** PWD. Normal texture and turgor without pallor or cyanosis. No petechiae or purpura
- **HEENT:**
  - **Head:** normocephalic without evidence of trauma. Fontanel normal (if still open)
  - **Eyes:** moist and bright. Sclera and conjunctiva normal. PERRLA. EOMIs. No nystagmus or diplopia noted
  - **Ears:** canals patent. TMs clear. No pre- or postauricular lymphadenopathy
  - **Nose:** patent without rhinorrhea or nasal flaring
  - **Mouth/Throat:** MMM. Posterior pharynx clear without lesions, erythema, or exudates
- **Neck:** FROM. Supple without meningismus or lymphadenopathy
- **Chest:** no retractions noted; no grunting or stridor. Good tidal volume. CTA; no wheezes, crackles, or rhonchi. SaO_2 _____%, which is within normal limits (if 95% or >)
- **Heart:** RRR, no murmurs, rubs, or gallops
- **Abd:** soft, nondistended, BSA, NT. No masses or organomegaly palpated
- **Back:** without spinal or CVAT
- **GU:** normal external genitalia without rash. No hernia noted
- **Extremities:** FROM. Good strength bilaterally. Neurovascular intact. No cyanosis or edema
- **Neuro:** alert, active, and developmentally normal for age. GCS 15. Muscle tone good and equal, bilaterally. No focal neurological findings noted or abnormal neuro findings noted

(cont.)

SYNCOPE (cont.)

⊙ TIPS

- Syncope during exercise associated with a systolic ejection murmur requires emergency cardiology consultation
- Always obtain an EKG after a syncopal episode

DON'T MISS!

- Always inquire about family history of cardiac disease and sudden death

SEIZURES

Febrile seizures are the most common cause of seizures in children from **6 months to 5 years** of age with an incidence of 2% to 5%. The actual etiology of febrile seizures is not well understood; benign, simple febrile seizures are likely influenced by genetic and familial factors. Risk factors include males, children who are developmentally delayed or have underlying neurological impairment, and family history of febrile seizures. Generally accepted criteria for febrile seizures include **temperature >38°C** and no evidence of neurological infection or inflammation, systemic disease, or metabolic dysfunction that may also cause seizures. An accurate rectal temperature <38°C should raise concern for other seizure causes

SEIZURE CLASSIFICATIONS

- **Simple (benign) febrile seizure:** generalized clonic or clonic–tonic seizure lasting <15 minutes. The child is healthy and neurologically intact before and after the seizure. No evidence that fever or seizure was caused by an infectious disease such as meningitis or encephalitis. As many as 1/3 of children with a simple febrile seizure will experience a recurrence
- **Complex febrile seizure:** prolonged > 15 minutes or more than one seizure in 24 hours. May have focal neurological signs at time of seizure or in postictal period such as transient weakness of an extremity (Todd's paresis) or clonic movements of only one extremity or side of body
- **Symptomatic febrile seizure:** preexisting neurologic abnormality or acute illness

(cont.)

SEIZURES (cont.)

PE

Physical examination findings reveal a neurologically and developmentally healthy child and no signs of meningitis or encephalitis (e.g., stiff neck or persistent mental status changes)

- **General:** alert, active, drowsy, sleepy, ill, or toxic appearing
- **VS and SAO$_2$:** note VS and interpret as normal or abnormal, SaO$_2$ interpretation, weight in kg
- **Skin:** PWD, normal texture and turgor; no cyanosis. No petechiae or purpura
- **HEENT:**
  - **Head:** normocephalic without evidence of trauma. Fontanel normal (if still open)
  - **Eyes:** moist and bright. Sclera and conjunctiva normal. Pupils are equal, round, and reactive to light. EOMI or tracks normally. No nystagmus or diplopia noted
  - **Ears:** TMs and canals patent. No pre- or postauricular erythema or lymphadenopathy
  - **Nose:** patent without rhinorrhea or nasal flaring
  - **Face:** normal strength and sensation; no asymmetry
  - **Mouth/Throat:** MMM. Posterior pharynx clear without lesions, erythema, or exudate
- **Neck:** FROM, supple without meningismus or nuchal rigidity, no lymphadenopathy
- **Chest:** no retractions noted; no grunting or stridor. Good tidal volume. Lungs clear to auscultation; no wheezes, crackles, or rhonchi. SaO$_2$ _____%, which is within normal limits (if 95% or >)
- **Heart:** RRR, no murmurs, rubs, or gallops. Normal S1 and S2
- **Abd:** soft, nondistended. BSA, NT, no masses or organomegaly
- **Back:** no spinal or CVAT
- **GU:** normal external genitalia without rash. No hernia noted
- **Extremities:** FROM, good strength bilaterally. Neurovascularly intact. No cyanosis or edema
- **Neuro:** alert, active, and developmentally normal for age with normal behavior. GCS 15. Muscle tone good and equal, bilaterally. No focal neurological findings noted or mental status changes

MDM/DDx

Initial efforts should be a detailed history and physical examination focused on identification of the **cause of fever**, which can be precipitated by either **viral or bacterial infections.** **Meningitis** is a priority differential diagnosis in any child who presents with fever, and a lumbar puncture may be indicated based on clinical suspicion or the presence of meningeal signs. A lumbar puncture should also be considered in young children (6–12 months) with unclear or not up-to-date immunizations for *Haemophilus influenzae* type b (hib) or *Streptococcus pneumoniae*. Children who are on antibiotics for another focal infection may require a lumbar puncture as the antibiotics can mask the clinical findings of meningitis. A history of **recent DPT or MMR vaccination** should also be investigated

(cont.)

SEIZURES (cont.)

MANAGEMENT

The **only essential workup** for most simple febrile seizures is a **careful HX and physical exam** that will confirm the Dx and R/O other more serious etiologies

Labs

- No specific studies are indicated for a simple febrile seizure. Other lab tests may be indicated by the nature of the underlying febrile illness and include: CBC with diff, chem panel, blood culture, UA, and culture

Lumbar Puncture

- Signs and SXS of bacterial meningitis:
    - May be minimal or absent in children < 12 months
    - Subtle in children 12 to 18 months
    - >18 months, decision to perform LP is based on clinical suspicion of meningitis

Imaging

- CXR if respiratory symptoms present
- CT and MRI are not indicated in pts with simple febrile seizures

Other

- EEG is not indicated in children with simple febrile seizures

Medications

- Antipyretics for comfort
- **Seizure control for seizures lasting >5 minutes:**
    - Lorazepam IV or IM (0.05–0.1 mg/kg)
    - Midazolam IM (0.2 mg/kg)
    - Diazepam IV or PR (0.2–0.5 mg/kg)

(cont.)

SEIZURES (cont.)

DOCUMENTATION/DICTATION

- **General:** well-developed well-nourished child who is awake and active. Interacts appropriately with surroundings and examiner, in no acute distress
- **VS and SaO$_2$:** note VS and interpret as normal or abnormal, SaO$_2$ interpretation, weight in kg
- **Skin:** pink, warm, and dry. Normal texture and turgor without pallor or cyanosis. No petechiae or purpura
- **HEENT:**
  - **Head:** normocephalic without evidence of trauma. Fontanel normal (if still open)
  - **Eyes:** moist and bright. Sclera and conjunctiva normal. PERRLA. EOMIs. No nystagmus or diplopia noted
  - **Ears:** canals patent. TMs clear. No pre- or postauricular lymphadenopathy
  - **Nose:** patent without rhinorrhea or nasal flaring
  - **Mouth/Throat:** MMM. Posterior pharynx clear without lesions, erythema, or exudates
- **Neck:** FROM. Supple without meningismus or lymphadenopathy
- **Chest:** no retractions noted; no grunting or stridor. Good tidal volume. CTA; no wheezes, crackles, or rhonchi. SaO$_2$ _____%, which is within normal limits (if 95% or >)
- **Heart:** RRR, no murmurs, rubs, or gallops
- **Abd:** soft, nondistended. No apparent tenderness. No masses or organomegaly palpated. BSA
- **Back:** without spinal or CVAT
- **GU:** normal external genitalia without rash. No hernia noted
- **Extremities:** FROM. Good strength bilaterally. Neurovascularly intact. No cyanosis or edema
- **Neuro:** alert, active, and developmentally normal for age. GCS 15. Muscle tone good and equal, bilaterally. No focal neurological findings noted

❯ TIP

- EEG is not indicated in children with simple febrile seizures

DON'T MISS!

- Signs and SXS of bacterial meningitis can be subtle or absent in children esp. <12 months; decision to perform LP is based on clinical suspicion of meningitis

DIABETIC KETOACIDOSIS

HX

- Classic symptoms of DKA often absent in toddlers
- Insidious onset of somewhat vague symptoms
- Fatigue and malaise, weight loss
- F/C, N/V, abd pain, polydipsia, polyuria, polyphagia
- PMH: DM, compliance with insulin regimens, use of insulin pump, name of endocrinologist
- FH: DM
- SH: ETOH, tobacco, illicit drugs
- Tolerating PO, appetite, fluid intake, wet diapers, BM
- LNMP
- Meds (e.g., insulin pump use)
- Immunizations
- Allergies

PE

- **General:** alert, malaise, weak, toxic appearing
- **VS and SaO$_2$:** fever, hyperventilation/Kussmaul respirations, tachycardia, hypotension, pulse ox, delayed cap refill
- **Skin:** PWD or pale, cool, moist; sunken eyes, tenting of skin, dry mucous membranes, dehydration, delayed
- **HEENT:**
  - **Eyes:** pupils PERRLA and EOMI
  - **Ears:** TMs and canals clear
  - **Nose:** patent
  - **Mouth/Throat:** MMM or acetone odor on breath (ketosis)
- **Neck:** supple, no lymphadenopathy, no meningismus, no JVD
- **Chest:** CTA bilaterally
- **Heart:** RRR, no murmur, gallop, rub; clear tones. Tachypnea or hyperventilation (Kussmaul respirations) or tachycardia with DKA
- **Abd:** soft/flat/distended; BSA, guarding, rebound (jump up and down), rigid, tender, pulsatile masses, hernia
- **Back:** NT
- **Extremities:** FROM
- **Neuro:** AMS without evidence of head trauma

MDM/DDx

Diabetic ketoacidosis is a complex metabolic state of hyperglycemia, ketosis, and acidemia; result of absolute or relative deficiency of insulin in type 1 or type 2 DM. Approximately 25% of newly diagnosed pts with type 1 diabetes mellitus present with an acute **infection**. Bimodal age peaks at 4 to 6 years and again at 10 to 14 years. Possible poor compliance with insulin regimen or parent/pt may lack competence. Insulin pump failure is also a common cause. DKA can result in a significant fluid volume deficit and correction of **fluid and electrolyte imbalance**, which is the mainstay of treatment. There is a potentially life-threatening low total-body potassium level with DKA that can lead to **cardiac dysrhythmias**; close monitoring is required. Pt may also have underlying endocrine changes of adolescence (thelarche, adrenarche, menarche). Other conditions that should be considered in children include other causes of **metabolic acidosis, UTI, pneumonia, sepsis, dehydration, AGE**.

(cont.)

DIABETIC KETOACIDOSIS (cont.)

MANAGEMENT

- **ABCs, venous access,** immediate identification by **FSBG,** NPO
- **Volume resuscitation:** NS bolus 20 mL/kg over 30 to 60 minutes followed by 10 mL/kg bolus over next 60 minutes. When VS stable, maintain volume according to weight; slower hydration over 48 hours associated with less risk of cerebral edema
- **Fluid maintenance guidelines:**
  - 0 to 12 kg: 80 mL/kg/24 hr
  - 2 to 20 kg: 65 mL/kg/24 hr
  - 20 to 35 kg: 55 mL/kg/24 hr
  - 35 to 60 kg: 45 mL/kg/24 hr
- **Hyperglycemia:** goal to decrease glucose level by no more than 100 mg/dL/hr; requires simultaneous correction of potassium deficit
- **Continuous low-dose regular insulin** infusion 0.1 U/kg/hr IV is safer than bolus; better control and gradual correction of hyperglycemia. Teens with insulin resistance may need >0.1 U/kg/hr. (Some experts recommend waiting 1 hour to administer insulin to decrease incidence of cerebral edema.)
- **Monitor glucose hourly** and add 5% or 10% dextrose to IV fluids when glucose drops to 250 to 300 mg/dL
- **Avoid hypoglycemia:** maintain glucose 50 to 150 mg/dL during insulin infusion. Continue insulin infusion until ketosis resolved (bicarbonate >18 mg/dL and pH >7.3) and subcutaneous insulin started
- **Potassium:** begin with isotonic fluid resuscitation. When potassium level <5 mEq/L and there is normal urine output, begin replacement. Monitor potassium at least every 1 to 2 hours and watch worsening acidosis. Potassium IV replacement guidelines (may also give PO or NG with rapid absorption):
  - <2.5 mEq/L: 1 mEq per kg of weight infused over 1 hour
  - 2.5 to 3.5 mEq/L: 40 mEq/L
  - 3.5 to 5.5 mEq/L: 20 mEq/L
- **Acidosis:** IV fluid replacement and insulin will correct acidosis. Sodium bicarbonate not required and contraindicated in most cases
- **Labs:** CBC with diff, chem panel; serum ketone, lactate, osmolality levels; phosphate and magnesium; UA (glucose, ketone, osmolality) and UCG; appropriate cultures; ABG/VBG. Possible toxicology screen
  - In known diabetic, elevated high glycosylated hemoglobin (HbA1c) indicates poor insulin compliance
- **EKG:** hyperkalemia causes peaked T waves and cardiac dysrhythmias
- **Imaging:** CXR for infiltrate; CT brain for cerebral edema
- **Meds:** if bacterial infection is suspected, empiric Abx coverage for suspected etiology
  - Antiemetics if needed
- **Admit**
- **Consult:** pediatric endocrinology consultation

(cont.)

DIABETIC KETOACIDOSIS (cont.)

DICTATION/DOCUMENTATION

- **General:** level of activity and interaction, distress. Strong cry. Lethargic
- **VS and SaO$_2$:** afebrile, tachycardia, tachypnea, hypotension
- **Skin:** PWD, normal texture and turgor, no cyanosis or pallor, appears well hydrated; no rash
- **HEENT:**
    - **Head:** normocephalic. Fontanel (anterior and posterior) flat, full, or bulging
    - **Eyes:** sclera white and conjunctivae pink. PERRLA, EOMIs
    - **Ears:** canals and TMs normal, no pre- or postauricular lymphadenopathy or erythema
    - **Nose:** mucosa pink and patent, without rhinorrhea or nasal flaring
    - **Mouth/Throat:** MMM, posterior pharynx clear without lesions, erythema, exudate, or asymmetry
- **Neck:** supple, FROM, no meningismus, torticollis, or lymphadenopathy
- **Chest:** no tachypnea, retractions, or accessory muscle use. Lungs clear to auscultation; no wheezes, rales, or rhonchi
- **Heart:** RRR, no murmurs, rubs, or gallops
- **Abd:** BSA, soft, nondistended. NT. No masses or hepatosplenomegaly.
- **Back:** no spinal or CVAT
- **Extremities:** FROM, good strength and tone bilaterally. Neurovascular intact
- **Neuro:** alert, active, with age-appropriate behavior, GCS 15, no focal neurological findings noted

⊙ TIPS

- Possible poor compliance with insulin regimen or parent/pt may lack competence
- Insulin pump failure may also lead to DKA
- Monitor closely during fluid administration; cerebral edema is the leading cause of death in DKA

DON'T MISS!

Subtle signs and SXS of DKA:
- Fatigue, malaise, F/C, weight loss
- N/V, abd pain
- Polydipsia, polyuria, polyphagia

SICKLE CELL DISEASE

HX

- Recent stressor or trigger for vaso-occlusive crisis: exposure to hot or cold weather, hypoxemia, infection, dehydration, ETOH/illicit drug use, pregnancy, exertional stress
- New-onset jaundice <1 year
- Sudden onset of body or joint pain
- Nonspecific abd or low back pain
- Swelling of hands and feet
- F/C, nonspecific vomiting
- CP, shortness of breath (SOB), wheezing, cough, asthma attack, feeling faint
- Altered mental status
- Priapism
- Hematuria
- Soft tissue infection or ulcerations
- Infants: poor feeding, lethargic, irritable
- Neck pain, stiffness
- Inguinal pain, painful weight bearing
- Decreased stamina for physical activity
- HX of aplastic crises or change in chronic pain pattern and frequency
- PMH: anemia, SCD, pulmonary HTN, acute chest syndrome, CVA, aplastic crisis, splenic sequestration, hospitalizations
- Meds/allergies

PE

- **General:** position of pt, level of distress, toxic appearing; underweight or evidence of growth retardation
- **VS and SAO$_2$:** fever, tachycardia, hypoxia
- **Skin:** PWD, or pallor, cyanosis mottling. Icterus/jaundice; erythema or edema of extremities or joints. Petechiae, purpura, vesicles. Scaling, blistering, peeling
- **HEENT:**
    - **Head:** normocephalic, atraumatic
    - **Eyes:** sclera and conjunctivae normal, icterus, ptosis; PERRLA, EOMI. Fundi: retinal vascular changes, proliferative retinitis
    - **Ears:** canals and TMs normal
    - **Nose:** rhinorrhea or nasal flaring
    - **Face:** slapped-cheek appearance; symmetrical strength and sensation
    - **Mouth/Throat:** MMM, posterior pharynx clear, no erythema, exudate
- **Neck:** supple, meningismus, lymphadenopathy
- **Chest:** no retractions or accessory muscle use; CTA without wheezes, rhonchi, crackles; normal TV; NT to palpation
- **Heart:** RRR, no murmur, gallop, rub; tones clear
- **Abd:** soft, BSA, NT to palp, guarding, rebound, rigidity, distention. No HSM, neg Murphy's sign
- **GU:** normal external genitalia; no priapism
- **Back:** no spinal or CVAT
- **Extremities:** atraumatic, NT to palp; moves all extrems with good strength, distal neurovascularly intact with good pulses
- **Neuro:** alert and oriented, GCS 15, focal neuro deficits, speech clear, gait steady. Neg Brudzinski/Kernig signs

(cont.)

SICKLE CELL DISEASE (cont.)

MDM/DDx

Sickle cell trait affects one in 12 African Americans in the United States; having the gene or trait rarely causes **sickle cell disease** (SCD). SCD is a serious inherited disease that causes hemolysis and tissue hypoxia and affects various organs. SCD usually manifests early in childhood; infants <6 months are protected by fetal hemoglobin, which is not affected by the sickle cell gene. SCD is the most common inherited blood disorder in the United States; affecting more than 70,000 people. One in about every 500 African Americans is affected; less commonly Hispanics. Other groups include individuals with African–Caribbean, Asian, or Mediterranean background. Pts most commonly present with an episodic pain crisis or **vaso-occlusive crisis** caused by sickling cells that obstruct the microcirculation. **Dactylitis** is a hand–foot syndrome that affects toddlers and causes hands and feet to become painful and swollen. As the child grows, long bones are more affected. Consider **avascular necrosis** of the femoral or humeral head with complaint of joint pain. Long-bone pain may be caused by **bone marrow infarction**. Fever with cough, chest pain, and SOB raises concern for **pneumonia** or **ACS; asthma** significantly increases risk for acute chest syndrome.

Signs of **acute abdomen** are often severe and may be caused by organ infarction. The spleen can trap or sequester enough blood to cause hypovolemia and shock. Acute abd pain with rapid splenomegaly and elevated reticulocyte count may indicate life-threatening **splenic sequestration;** major cause of mortality <5 years. Pts with abd pain and distention may have a reactive **ileus**. Incidence of **cholelithiasis** in children with SCD is 50% and often occurs before 10 years of age. Acute **mesenteric ischemia** or **perforation** must also be considered. **Anemia** is chronic and hemolytic and usually well tolerated. Infection with usually benign parvovirus B-19 can lead to **aplastic crisis** because it affects bone marrow and causes a rapid reduction in Hgb without adequate reticulocytosis. Aplastic crisis can also be precipitated by folic acid deficiency. The crisis is self-limited and resolves in 1 to 2 weeks as the bone marrow recovers. Sickling and chronic RBC damage eventually lead to splenic damage and result in functional asplenia, making children very susceptible to **infections** such as strep **pneumonia, meningitis, and osteomyelitis**. Infections are the leading cause of death; sepsis risk is greatest <3 years. Other diseases that may have a similar presentation include RA, hemolytic anemia, Legg–Calve–Perthes Dx, PE, and septic joint

MANAGEMENT

- Supplemental O$_2$ (indicated only if hypoxic)
- **Hydration:** IV D5 1/2 NS hydration; rapid bolus NS 20 mL/kg if dehydrated or shock
- **Labs:** CBC with diff (anemia; left shift), T&S/T&C, reticulocyte count (>0.5%); chem panel, LFTs; UA (RBCs w/o casts or pyuria indicate papillary necrosis), UCG. Possible cultures and LP if febrile or altered; ABG/VBG
- **Imaging:** CXR if cough or febrile. Plain films of painful extremity or joint; MRI may be needed to clarify bone infection or infarct. CT/MRI brain to R/O stroke. Abd ultz if concern for cholecystitis or cholelithiasis. Pelvic ultz for ectopic pregnancy. MRI to detect bone marrow infarction, marrow hyperplasia, osteomyelitis, and osteonecrosis
- **EKG:** indicated for chest pain, abnormal pulse rate, palpitations, or syncope
- **Transfusion:** Hgb <10 and in acute crisis or <6 with low reticulocyte count; aplastic crisis or splenic sequestration. Infuse 10 mL/kg PRBCs to return to baseline Hgb
- **Consult:** cardiology, neurology, urology (priapism)
- **Admission:** acute chest syndrome, sepsis, or serious infection, aplastic crisis, uncontrolled pain, WBC >30 or platelets <100

SICKLE CELL DISEASE (cont.)

MEDS

- Nonsteroidal analgesics (e.g., ketorolac, ASA, APAP, ibuprofen)
- Opioid analgesics (e.g., oxycodone/ASA, methadone, morphine sulfate, oxycodone/APAP, fentanyl, nalbuphine, codeine, APAP/codeine)
- Empiric Abx for suspected infection or identified focal infections (e.g., cefuroxime, amoxicillin/clavulanate, PVK, ceftriaxone, azithromycin, cefaclor)
- Antimetabolites: hydroxyurea
- Folic acid

DICTATION/DOCUMENTATION

- **General:** awake and alert, in no obvious distress
- **VS and SaO$_2$:** afebrile, no tachycardia, tachypnea, or hypoxemia
- **Skin:** PWD, no jaundice, cyanosis, or pallor; no petechiae or purpura. No evidence of soft tissue infection
- **HEENT:**
  - **Head:** normocephalic
  - **Eyes:** PERRLA, sclera and conjunctivae clear; no icterus
  - **Ears:** canals and TMs normal
  - **Nose:** patent
  - **Mouth/Throat:** MMM, posterior pharynx clear
- **Neck:** supple, no meningismus or lymphadenopathy
- **Chest:** NT, no orthopnea or dyspnea noted; no retractions or accessory muscle use. CTA bilaterally, no wheezes, rhonchi, crackles
- **Heart:** RRR, no murmur, gallop, rub; tones clear
- **Abd:** BSA, soft, NT, no guarding, rebound, rigidity. No HSM
- **Back:** no spinal or CVAT
- **Extremities:** no asymmetry or deformity. Moves all extrems well. No swelling, edema, tenderness; no joint irritability. Normal neurovascular status
- **Neuro:** alert, GCS 15, no focal neuro deficits noted. Normal reflexes; neg Babinski

◐ TIP

- Do not transfuse higher than baseline Hgb to avoid heart failure or stroke

DON'T MISS!

- Splenic sequestration: sudden enlargement of spleen with drop in Hgb 2 g/dL and increase in reticulocytes
- Acute chest syndrome: fever, cough, wheezing, SOB, chest pain, and infiltrate
- Aplastic crisis with low reticulocyte count
- Signs of sepsis or shock
- Biliary etiology versus vaso-occlusive in acute abd pain

HEMATOLOGIC/ONCOLOGIC DISORDERS

HX

- General appearance, LOC, weight loss
- Onset
- Location/distribution and progression
- Duration
- Characteristics: mucous membrane involvement, palmer/sole involvement
- Itching, burning, painful skin
- Pallor, rash, jaundice
- N/V/F/C, myalgias, arthralgias
- HA, runny nose, sore throat, cough, wheezing
- Limp, bone pain
- Night sweats, swollen glands, swelling/edema
- New-onset seizure, paresthesias
- Possible exposures (e.g., meds, personal care products, recreation, travel, food)
- FH: Heme/oncologic disorders
- SH: Sick contacts, travel
- Allergies/Immunizations/Meds

PE

- **General:** awake, alert, age-appropriate behavior, well versus toxic appearing
- **VS and SaO$_2$:** febrile
- **Skin:** PWD or lesions—location/distribution—generalized, localized, dermatomal, discrete, diffuse, confluent, grouped, annular, linear, discoid. Color and temperature of lesions—erythema, blanching, petechiae, ecchymosis
- **HEENT:**
  - **Head:** normocephalic, atraumatic, kerion, scaly patches, hair loss
  - **Eyes:** PERRLA, EOMI, sclera and conjunctivae clear/icteric, periorbital lesions, STS, or erythema
  - **Ears:** canals and TMs normal, pre- or postauricular lymphadenopathy
  - **Nose:** normal, rhinorrhea. Vesicle at tip of nose (Hutchinson sign), concern for ophthalmic HZV
  - **Face:** symmetric, "slapped cheeks" lesions
  - **Mouth/Throat:** MMM; dry, cracked lips; posterior pharynx clear; mucosal lesions' strawberry tongue; palatine petechiae; vesicles; Koplik spots; gingival hypertrophy
- **Neck:** supple, FROM, lymphadenopathy or meningismus
- **Chest:** CTA, heart sounds
- **Abd:** BSA, NT, HSM
- **Back:** spinal or CVAT
- **Extremities:** FROM with good strength
- **Neuro:** alert, GCS 15, no focal neuro deficits

MDM/DDx

Children with heme/onc disorders can present with **coagulopathy, DIC, factor deficiencies, ITP, platelet disorders, protein deficiencies, thromboembolism, von Willebrand disease, disorders of lymphocytic function** (combined b-cell or t-cell disorders, pure b-cell disorders), **heme synthesis disorders** (porphyria), **immune system disorders** (eosinophilia neutropenia, neutrophilia, splenomegaly), **lymphoproliferative disorders** (e.g., lymphoma), **plasma cell disorders** (e.g., multiple myeloma), **red blood cell disorders** (e.g., anemia, beta thalassemia, bone marrow failure, stem cell), **transfusion issues** (transfusion reactions or transfusion-transmitted diseases), or **uncommon red blood cell membrane disorders.**

(cont.)

HEMATOLOGIC/ONCOLOGIC DISORDERS (cont.)

MANAGEMENT

Labs

- CBC with manual diff, chem panel, platelets, UA/UCG, lactate, LDH, uric acid, LFTs, coags (assess for DIC), urine and blood culture if febrile
- EKG and echocardiography

Imaging

- CXR to evaluate for mediastinal mass
- Ultz
- LP as indicated
- Consults as indicated

DICTATION/DOCUMENTATION

- **General:** awake and alert, in no obvious distress. Not toxic appearing, no lethargy
- **VS and SaO₂:** afebrile, tachycardia, tachypnea, hypotension
- **Skin:** PWD, normal texture and turgor, no cyanosis or pallor, appears well hydrated; no rash. Mucous membrane involvement, blisters, peeling, extensive erythema, presence or absence of purpura/petechiae, or secondary infection. Describe rash or lesions, including location, distribution, and configuration
- **HEENT:**
  - **Head:** normocephalic
  - **Eyes:** PERRLA, EOMI, sclera and conjunctiva clear
  - **Ears:** canals and TMs normal
  - **Nose:** patent
  - **Mouth/Throat:** MMM, posterior pharynx clear
- **Neck:** supple. FROM, no JVD, trachea midline, no bruits
- **Chest:** no tachypnea or dyspnea noted; no retractions or accessory muscle use. Lungs clear bilaterally, no wheezes, rhonchi, or crackles
- **Heart:** RRR, no murmur, gallop, rub; tones clear
- **Abd:** soft, BSA, NT, no epigastric tenderness, mass
- **Back:** no CVAT
- **Extremities:** no swelling, edema, tenderness
- **Neuro:** alert, GCS 15, no focal neuro deficits

⊙ TIP

- All pts with suspected fever of unknown origin and other SXS (e.g., neutropenia) should be referred to peds heme/oncology specialist

DON'T MISS!

- Fever and neutropenia
- Manual differential for identification of blast cells
- Life-threatening conditions associated with hyperleukocytosis, tumor lysis syndrome, or sepsis

TOXICOLOGIC DISORDERS

HX

- Toxin or ingested substance; route, when exposed or ingested
- Concern for ingestion or witnessed
- Concern for abuse, neglect, child maltreatment
- Changes in appearance and behavior—malaise, lethargy, restlessness, irritability, ALOC
- F/C, N/V/D
- Gagging, choking, cough, rash
- Sweating or hot, dry skin; rash
- Muscle weakness, spasm, twitching
- Possible exposure to adult medication; visits to other households; what medications available, especially TCA
- Home remedies for illness or pain
- Possible exposure to plants
- LNMP
- Social HX: HEADSS (Home, Education/Employment, Activities, Drugs, Sexuality, Suicide/Depression)
- Meds
- Allergies/Immunizations
- Maltreatment/Munchhausen's syndrome by proxy

PE

- **General**: position of pt, level of distress, alert, agitated, lethargic, comatose
- **VS and SaO$_2$**: fever, tachycardia or bradycardia, hypotension
- **Skin**: PWD, moist, pale, rashes or lesions, jaundice, pallor, cyanosis
- **HEENT:**
  - **Head**: AT, normocephalic
  - **Eyes**: sclera and conjunctiva, tearing, PERRLA, EOMI, nystagmus, ptosis, diplopia
  - **Ears**: canals and TM clear
  - **Nose**: patent, drainage
  - **Face**: symmetry, strength, sensation
  - **Mouth/Throat**: MMM, drooling, stridor, posterior pharynx clear; odors on breath
- **Neck**: supple, FROM, meningismus, lymphadenopathy
- **Chest**: accessory muscle use, retractions; CTA, wheezes, rhonchi, crackles
- **Heart**: RRR, no murmur, gallop, rub, clear tones
- **Abd**: flat, BS decreased or hyperactive; tenderness, masses, organomegaly
- **Back**: spinal or CVAT
- **Extremities**: FROM, weakness, paresthesias, distal CMS, ataxia
- **Neuro**: A&O × 3, GCS 15, no focal neuro deficits. Speech, gait, ataxia

(cont.)

TOXICOLOGIC DISORDERS (cont.)

MDM/DDx

Most pediatric ingestions involve nontoxic substances and most involve children < 6 years. Older children are at risk for more serious or intentional ingestions. The priority for possible **accidental** or **intentional toxic exposures (maltreatment/Munchhausen's syndrome by proxy)** is to maintain ABCs and identify etiology. Assessment of VS, skin signs, pupils, lung and bowel sounds, and neuro status can help provide important clues to specific poisonings. Elevated temperature can be caused by **TCA, phenothiazine,** or **antihistamine ingestion. Anesthetic agents** can cause life-threatening **malignant hyperthermia.** The anticholinergic effects on these pts often include tachycardia, HTN, agitation with dilated pupils, and hot, dry skin. **Sedatives, ETOH,** and **sympatholytic medications** (e.g., clonidine) can cause decreased respiratory rate or effort and may lead to hypotension and AMS. **Illicit use of methamphetamine, cocaine,** or **ketamine** can cause a sympathomimetic response that can lead to significant tachycardia and HTN and is often associated with increased muscle activity, agitation, psychotic behaviors, mydriasis, and diaphoresis. Other substances causing pts to present with increased agitation are **PCP, LSD, MAOI,** and **lithium.** The classic **organophosphate toxicity** is a cholinergic crisis (SLUDGE) that includes salivation, lacrimation, urination, defecation, GI disturbances, and emesis. Pts can be lethargic, diaphoretic, have muscle twitching/fasciculations, weakness, bronchospasm, and increased BS.

MANAGEMENT

- **Poison control consultation with simultaneous maintenance of ABCs**
- Attempt to identify toxin, and remove if possible
- Oxygen/Intubation as indicated (GCS < 8)
- IV access and fluid resuscitation if needed. FSBG
- **Labs**—CBC with diff, chem panel (anion gap), ETOH, UA/UCG, tox screen
- **Cardiac:** monitor, EKG; treat arrhythmias
- **Imaging:** CXR, CT
- **Toxin(s):** decontamination measures as indicated; remove from skin, lavage as indicated; antidote, if available—possibly activated charcoal
- **Consults** as needed
- **Admit:** ICU for severe cardiac or neuro toxicity, and any suspected or confirmed TCA cyclic overdose requires 12 to 24 hours of cardiac monitoring. Telemetry admission for cardiac monitoring if no evidence of serious CNS or cardiac involvement for signs of anticholinergic toxicity: resting tachycardia, mydriasis, agitation/lethargy, hyperthermia
- **Asymptomatic pts:** screen for suicidal intent; observe at least 8 hours or admit to psych facility

DICTATION/DOCUMENTATION

- Specific to type of ingestion—CNS toxic, cardiotoxic (see "Pain"/"Fever"/ "Maltreatment"/"Chest Pain"/"Abd Pain"/"Seizures")

● TIPS

- Report child abuse, neglect, or child maltreatment if concern for inadequate supervision or Münchausen syndrome by proxy suspected
- Screen for suicidal behavior and admit to a psych facility, if indicated, when medically stable

(cont.)

TOXICOLOGIC DISORDERS (cont.)

DON'T MISS!

- Potentially fatal single-dose ingestion (even very small amounts such as one tablet) including but not limited to:
  - Antidepressants: TCAs (imipramine, amitriptyline, desipramine), MAOIs
  - Antimalarials
  - Antipsychotics
  - Cardiovascular: clonidine, verapamil, nifedipine
  - Drugs of abuse: ETOH, amphetamines, opioids/sedatives/hypnotics, LSD, nicotine (one whole cigarette can be fatal); consider methadone

- Others: small but excessive amount of 2% viscous lidocaine, hypoglycemic medications, colchicine, Lomotil, iron, ASA, cold medications containing pseudoephedrine, OTC and topical medications, or preparations such as oil of wintergreen. In addition to common cleaning agents, household items to consider are alcohols, gasoline, lighter fluid, and motor oil. Some plants are also potentially fatal such as toxic mushrooms, apricot seeds, or plants used in home remedies

INDEX